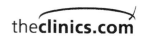

CLINICS IN PODIATRIC MEDICINE AND SURGERY

Surgical Reconstruction of the High-Risk Patient

GUEST EDITOR
Thomas S. Roukis, DPM, FACFAS

CONSULTING EDITOR
Thomas Zgonis, DPM, FACFAS

October 2008 • Volume 25 • Number 4

SAUNDERS

An Imprint of Elsevier, Inc.
PHILADELPHIA   LONDON   TORONTO   MONTREAL   SYDNEY   TOKYO

W.B. SAUNDERS COMPANY
A Division of Elsevier Inc.

1600 John F. Kennedy Blvd., Suite 1800, Philadelphia, PA 19103-2899

http://www.theclinics.com

CLINICS IN PODIATRIC MEDICINE
AND SURGERY
October 2008
Editor: Patrick Manley

Volume 25, Number 4
ISSN 0891-8422
ISBN-13: 978-1-4160-6342-1
ISBN-10: 1-4160-6342-0

Reprints. For copies of 100 or more of articles in this publication, please contact the Commercial Reprints Department, Elsevier Inc., 360 Park Avenue South, New York, NY 10010-1710. Tel.: 212-633-3812; Fax: 212-462-1935; E-mail: reprints@elsevier.com.

Clinics in Podiatric Medicine and Surgery (ISSN 0891-8422) is published quarterly by Elsevier Inc., 360 Park Avenue South, New York, NY 10010-1710. Months of publication are January, April, July, and October. Business and Editorial Offices: 1600 John F. Kennedy Blvd., Suite 1800, Philadelphia, PA 191023-2899. Customer Service Office: 6277 Sea Harbor Drive, Orlando, FL 32887-4800. Periodicals postage paid at New York, NY, and additional mailing offices. Subscription prices are $208.00 per year for US individuals, $327.00 per year for US institutions, $107.00 per year for US students and residents, $250.00 per year for Canadian individuals, $396.00 for Canadian institutions, $279.00 for international individuals, $396.00 per year for international institutions and $143.00 per year for Canadian and foreign students/residents. To receive student/resident rate, orders must be accompanied by name of affiliated institution, date of term, and the *signature* of program/residency coordinator on institution letterhead. Orders will be billed at individual rate until proof of status is received. Foreign air speed delivery is included in all *Clinics* subscription prices. All prices are subject to change without notice. POSTMASTER: Send address changes to *Clinics in Podiatric Medicine and Surgery,* Elsevier Periodicals Customer Service, 6277 Sea Harbor Drive, Orlando, FL 32887-4800. **Customer Service: 1-800-654-2452 (US). From outside of the US, call 1-407-563-6020. Fax: 1-407-363-9661. E-mail: JournalsCustomerService-usa@elsevier.com.**

Clinics in Podiatric Medicine and Surgery is covered in *MEDLINE/PubMed (Index Medicus) and EMBASE/Excerpta Medica.*

Printed and bound by CPI Group (UK) Ltd, Croydon, CR0 4YY

Transferred to Digital Print 2011

CONSULTING EDITOR

THOMAS ZGONIS, DPM, FACFAS, Associate Professor, Department of Orthopaedic Surgery; Interim Chief, Division of Podiatric Medicine and Surgery; and Director, Reconstructive Foot and Ankle Surgery Fellowship, The University of Texas Health Science Center at San Antonio, San Antonio, Texas

GUEST EDITOR

THOMAS S. ROUKIS, DPM, FACFAS, Chief, Limb Preservation Service, Vascular/Endovascular Surgery Service; and Director, Limb Preservation Complex Lower Extremity Surgery and Research Fellowship, Limb Preservation Service, Vascular/Endovascular Surgery Service, Department of Surgery, Madigan Army Medical Center, Tacoma, Washington

CONTRIBUTORS

JEFFREY R. BAKER, DPM, AACFAS, Reconstructive Foot and Ankle Surgeon, Weil Foot and Ankle Institute, Des Plaines, Illinois; Attending Podiatric Surgeon, Weiss Memorial Hospital Podiatric Surgical Residency Program, Chicago, Illinois

GREGORIO CABAN, DPM, Attending Physician, Section of Podiatric Medicine and Surgery, Palmetto General Hospital, Hialeah, Florida

EMILY COOK, DPM, AACFAS, Clinical Instructor in Surgery, Harvard Medical School; and Harvard Podiatric Reconstruction and Research Fellow, Division of Podiatric Surgery, Department of Surgery, Beth Israel Deaconess Medical Center, Boston, Massachusetts

JEREMY COOK, DPM, AACFAS, Clinical Instructor in Surgery, Harvard Medical School; and Harvard Podiatric Reconstruction and Research Fellow, Division of Podiatric Surgery, Department of Surgery, Beth Israel Deaconess Medical Center, Boston, Massachusetts

LAWRENCE A. DIDOMENICO, DPM, FACFAS, Adjunct Professor, Ohio College of Podiatric Medicine; Director, Reconstructive Rearfoot and Ankle Surgical Fellowship, Ankle and Foot Care Centers, Ohio College of Podiatric Medicine, Independence, Ohio

JASON P. GLOVER, DPM, Reconstructive Foot and Ankle Surgeon, Rutherford Orthopaedics, Rutherfordton, North Carolina

LUKE C. JEFFRIES, DPM, AACFAS, Reconstructive Foot and Ankle Fellow and Clinical Instructor, Division of Podiatric Medicine and Surgery, Department of Orthopaedic Surgery, The University of Texas Health Science Center at San Antonio, San Antonio, Texas

ARMIN KOLLER, MD, Department of Technical Orthopaedics, Münster University Hospital, Northrhine-Westfalia, Germany

ADAM LANDSMAN, DPM, PhD, FACFAS, Associate Professor of Surgery, Harvard Medical School; and Division of Podiatric Surgery, Department of Surgery, Beth Israel Deaconess Medical Center, Boston, Massachusetts

LUIS E. MARIN, DPM, FACFAS, Residency Director, Podiatric Medicine and Surgery–36 Months Residency, Palmetto General Hospital, Hialeah, Florida

DENNIS B. McBROOM, DPM, Chief Resident, PGY-3, Podiatric Medicine and Surgery–36 Months Residency, Palmetto General Hospital, Hialeah, Florida

PATRICK A. McENEANEY, DPM, Third Year Podiatric Surgical Resident, Weiss Memorial Hospital Podiatric Surgical Residency Program, Chicago, Illinois

ALI ÖZNUR, MD, Associate Professor, Department of Orthopaedics and Traumatology, Hacettepe University, Sihhiye, Ankara, Turkey

ROBERTO H. RODRIGUEZ, DPM, AACFAS, Reconstructive Foot and Ankle Fellow and Clinical Instructor, Division of Podiatric Medicine and Surgery, Department of Orthopaedic Surgery, The University of Texas Health Science Center at San Antonio, San Antonio, Texas

THOMAS S. ROUKIS, DPM, FACFAS, Chief, Limb Preservation Service, Vascular/Endovascular Surgery Service; and Director, Limb Preservation Complex Lower Extremity Surgery and Research Fellowship, Limb Preservation Service, Vascular/Endovascular Surgery Service, Department of Surgery, Madigan Army Medical Center, Tacoma, Washington

VALERIE L. SCHADE, DPM, AACFAS, Fellow, Limb Preservation Complex Lower Extremity Surgery and Research Fellowship, Limb Preservation Service, Vascular/Endovascular Surgery Service, Department of Surgery, Madigan Army Medical Center, Tacoma, Washington

MONICA H. SCHWEINBERGER, DPM, AACFAS, Former Fellow, Limb Preservation Complex Lower Extremity Surgery and Research Fellowship; Limb Preservation Service, Vascular/Endovascular Surgery Service, Department of Surgery, Madigan Army Medical Center, MCHJ-SV, Tacoma, Washington

JOHN J. STAPLETON, DPM, AACFAS, Associate, Foot and Ankle Surgery, VSAS Orthopaedics, Lehigh Valley Hospital, Allentown; Clinical Assistant Professor of Surgery, Penn State College of Medicine, Hershey, Pennsylvania

THOMAS ZGONIS, DPM, FACFAS, Associate Professor, Department of Orthopaedic Surgery; Interim Chief, Division of Podiatric Medicine and Surgery; and Director, Reconstructive Foot and Ankle Surgery Fellowship, The University of Texas Health Science Center at San Antonio, San Antonio, Texas

CONTENTS

> Tendon lengthening and transfer are essential surgical procedures for every foot and ankle surgeon to master, because they are useful in restoring balance and correcting flexible foot deformities. These techniques are even more useful in treating the high-risk patient, because they involve minimal soft-tissue injury and maximum preservation of vascularity. The primary goal of this article is to supplement the foot and ankle surgeon's options for treating static and dynamic foot deformities in the high-risk patient by discussing useful tendon lengthening and transfer procedures about the forefoot, midfoot, and hindfoot.

> Soft-tissue ankle equinus contracture is an important component of numerous foot and ankle deformities. In high-risk patients who have multiple co-morbidities, procedure selection and careful surgical technique are paramount to increase the likelihood of postoperative success. This article discusses the indications for percutaneous Achilles tendon lengthening, open gastrocnemius recession, and endoscopic gastrocnemius recession, and provides a detailed

description of each surgical technique with pearls to avoid intra-perative and postoperative complications specific to the high-risk patient. Thorough knowledge of each of these techniques will aide the foot and ankle surgeon in appropriate peri-operative management of equinus deformity in a complex patient population.

This article focuses on minimal-incision metatarsal osteotomies for treating ulcerative lesions related to hallux valgus deformities and central and fifth metatarsal plantar ulcerations to correct the structural deformity responsible for the ulceration. The authors presented a structured review of the literature regarding complications associated with the use of minimum-incision surgical techniques available for the first, central, and fifth metatarsals and techniques to avoid them. Although a steep learning curve exists with these procedures, the advantage of performing minimum-incision metatarsal osteotomies in high-risk populations allows for rapid and predictable resolution of recalcitrant or recurrent ulcerations through correction of the underlying structural deformity with minimal complications.

Ray resection for localized necrosis, infection, and osteomyelitis is an accepted procedure allowing removal of the diseased toe and metatarsal. The traditional approach involves a rather lengthy incision and dissection that can compromise the vascular supply to the remaining forefoot. The use of minimum incision techniques to perform metatarsal ray resection as presented here represents a simple, reliable, and easily reproduced procedure that limits soft-tissue dissection and the associated wound healing-related complications inherent to the traditional approach. Following minimum incision metatarsal ray resection, the resultant defect from the toe amputation can be primarily closed, covered with a split-thickness skin graft, or closed in delayed primary fashion with the use of a mini-external fixation device. The authors present the proper indications and a step-by-step guide for performing minimum incision metatarsal ray resection with and without the supplemental use of mini-external fixation to close the soft-tissue defect about the toe amputation site.

Soft-tissue and osseous balancing of forefoot and midfoot amputations is imperative to provide the patient with a stable, durable, and functional residual foot. This article discusses reproducible methods for balancing transmetatarsal and Lisfranc amputations in high-risk patients, with detailed explanations of the recommended surgical techniques. In addition to performing the appropriate procedures for the individual patient, careful attention to the perioperative management of this patient population, with a multidisciplinary approach, is mandatory for long-term success.

Internal Pedal Amputations

Armin Koller

Internal pedal amputation consists of resection of the metatarsals, midtarsal bones, or talus with preservation of the toes and soft-tissue envelope. Although used in the past for the treatment of tuberculosis within the pedal skeleton, internal pedal amputations have become almost forgotten, historical procedures. However, following internal pedal amputations of a diabetic patient, the foot undergoes significant contracture that results in a stable, functional, foreshortened residual foot capable of being protected in custom-molded shoe gear with external or in-shoe orthoses. The author presents the surgical approach and postoperative treatment regime for each form of internal pedal amputation, as well as "pearls" for success.

Minimally Invasive Soft-Tissue and Osseous Stabilization (MISOS) Technique for Midfoot and Hindfoot Deformities

Thomas S. Roukis

The surgical repair of unstable midfoot and hindfoot deformities in the high-risk patient remains a challenge with little guidance available in the literature. The author presents a proposed surgical intervention for midfoot and hindfoot deformities utilizing a minimally invasive soft-tissue and osseous stabilization (MISOS) approach. The article presents a detailed, step-by-step description of the procedure used for these difficult limb salvage cases.

Corrective Midfoot Osteotomies

John J. Stapleton, Lawrence A. DiDomenico, and Thomas Zgonis

Corrective midfoot osteotomies involve complete separation of the forefoot and hindfoot through the level of the midfoot, followed by uni-, bi-, or triplanar realignment and arthrodesis. This technique can be performed through various approaches; however, in the high-risk patient, percutaneous and minimum incision techniques are necessary to limit the potential of developing soft tissue injury. These master level techniques require extensive surgical experience and detailed knowledge of lower extremity biomechanics. The authors discuss preoperative clinical and radiographic evaluation, specific operative techniques used, and postoperative management for the high-risk patient undergoing corrective midfoot osteotomy.

FORTHCOMING ISSUES

RECENT ISSUES

ELSEVIER
SAUNDERS

Clin Podiatr Med Surg
25 (2008) xiii–xiv

CLINICS IN
PODIATRIC
MEDICINE AND
SURGERY

Foreword

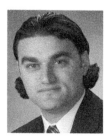

Thomas Zgonis, DPM, FACFAS
Consulting Editor

Being Thankful

It is with utmost pride, honor, and respect that I accept this position as the new Consulting Editor for the *Clinics in Podiatric Medicine and Surgery* starting with this issue of October 2008. It is certainly a big task and a new challenge that I have to face in my academic career. I must not forget, however, the people who have guided me early in my training and also helped me achieve my goals and education.

First, I want to thank Dr. Clinton Lowery and Drs. Nicki and Jeff Nigro from the University of Pittsburgh Medical Center in Pittsburgh, Pennsylvania, for accepting me into their residency program and showing me the early baby steps in my academic journey. After a solid residency, I moved on to a bigger step in my career by accepting a revisional and reconstructive foot and ankle surgery fellowship with Drs. Gary Peter Jolly and Peter Blume at the New Britain General Hospital, New Britain, Connecticut, affiliated with the Yale School of Medicine, New Haven, Connecticut. During that time, Dr. Jolly served as the president of the American College of Foot and Ankle Surgeons and essentially opened the doors to my educational, clinical, and surgical experience. In addition, Drs. Jolly and Blume always taught me the importance of academic medicine, research, and surgical excellence, and eventually, I was invited to accept a position as an Assistant Professor within the Department of Orthopaedics/Podiatry Division at The University of Texas Health Science Center (UTHSC) in San Antonio, Texas under the direct supervision of Dr. Lawrence Harkless. Dr. Harkless has been stellar in our profession for many years and personally helped me accomplish my goals within an academic institution. He has been a true leader and mentor and also guided me to establish and direct the current fellowships in research and reconstructive surgery at UTHSC in San Antonio, Texas.

Remembering and being thankful to all the people who have guided you throughout the most crucial steps in your career must be a certain appreciation and a lifetime recognition. So please, take a moment away from your busy daily schedule to thank your externship, residency, and fellowship directors along with all of the physicians and surgeons during your training, and appreciate the amount of time, dedication, passion, and extra work that they have had to perform for the advancement of the profession, education, and patient success. We seem to easily forget those who showed us the successful road in our profession in the face of our personal glory and maybe short-term success.

As a new Consulting Editor, I have made a strong initial step to make some changes under the direct guidance and help of our previous editor, Dr. Vincent Mandracchia. His long dedication to the *Clinics in Podiatric Medicine and Surgery* has been a tremendous asset to our profession and education and I am most grateful to him for my current position. I have added a national and international Editorial Board of prestigious foot and ankle experts to help us select and review the most current topics in the field of podiatric medicine and surgery. In addition, a new section, "Current Concepts and Techniques in Foot and Ankle Surgery," at the end of each issue encourages submissions from residents and fellows across the country and around the world.

In this issue, Dr. Roukis has been selected to serve as a guest editor for the "Surgical Reconstruction of the High-Risk Patient." He and his colleagues cover modern techniques, including percutaneous osseous and soft tissue procedures for the highly at-risk patient. In the presence of multiple comorbidities, peripheral vascular disease, and severe deformities, the minimally invasive percutaneous corrections have recently gained popularity in the literature. This issue will certainly become a great tool to guide you with the most difficult surgical candidates.

Finally, a great thank you to all of the Editorial Board members and to my wife Kristen and daughter Labrini for their understanding and support throughout this new challenge in my life.

Thomas Zgonis, DPM, FACFAS
Department of Orthopaedics/Podiatry Division
The University of Texas Health Science Center at San Antonio
7703 Floyd Curl Drive – MSC 7776
San Antonio, TX 78229

E-mail address: zgonis@uthscsa.edu

ELSEVIER
SAUNDERS

Clin Podiatr Med Surg
25 (2008) xv–xvii

CLINICS IN
PODIATRIC
MEDICINE AND
SURGERY

Preface

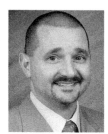

Thomas S. Roukis, DPM, FACFAS
Guest Editor

It is with great pleasure that I serve as guest editor for this issue of *Clinics in Podiatric Medicine and Surgery*, devoted to surgical reconstruction of the high-risk patient. The intent of this issue is to provide a step-by-step guideline for performing percutaneous and minimum incision soft-tissue and osseous reconstructive foot and ankle surgery techniques in patients with major deformity or traumatic injury with multiple medical comorbidities. This patient population will commonly have hostile tissues about the foot and ankle, making them at high risk for significant soft-tissue and osseous healing complications that could result in lower limb amputation. Therefore, minimizing the length and number of incisions and associated trauma to the soft-tissue envelope will lead to a greater likelihood of success postoperatively without compromising outcome. The authors selected are respected authorities on the topics they have been assigned and have graciously provided well-written and detailed articles for the reader's review.

Tenotomies and tendon transfers are frequently performed as adjunctive procedures during the global surgical correction of numerous foot and ankle deformities, but the myriad techniques and modifications available for the high-risk surgical patient have not been previously reported in a single article. Likewise, surgical procedures for correction of soft-tissue ankle equinus

The opinions or assertions contained herein are the private view of the author and are not to be construed as official or reflecting the views of the Department of the Army or the Department of Defense.

doi:10.1016/j.cpm.2008.05.011
podiatric.theclinics.com

are commonly discussed, but surprisingly little has been written about the actual performance of the procedures presented or clear guidance provided regarding "real world" indications and contraindications for each.

Minimum incision surgery about the forefoot took root in the podiatric community in the 1970s and 1980s. Regardless of whether these procedures will ever gain widespread acceptance by the foot and ankle community at large, minimum incision metatarsal osteotomies occasionally provide the only feasible means of performing structural, isolated, forefoot realignment in the high-risk patient in order to correct deformity resulting in ulceration. Similarly, minimal incision principles can be applied to performing metatarsal ray resections and represent a very elegant and effective approach that should become increasingly more popular as foot and ankle surgeons embrace this soft-tissue envelope protecting technique, as I have.

Balancing partial foot amputations through the use of various soft-tissue and osseous procedures is another commonly discussed topic, with surprisingly little written about the actual surgical techniques. The article presented in this issue of *Clinics* describes several effective procedures that are simple to perform and provide reproducible results. The concept of performing an "internal" transmetatarsal or midfoot amputation is intriguing and has certain benefits, beyond ease of acceptance by the patient, which are discussed in depth.

The performance of minimum incision soft-tissue and osseous surgery about the midfoot and hindfoot has received little attention in the medical literature and essentially no attention with regard to the high-risk foot, yet the procedures are extremely effective, with relatively few complications when performed properly. These techniques should be a part of every foot and ankle surgeon's procedure "tool-box." Likewise, the ability to successfully perform corrective midfoot osteotomies is an essential skill that every foot and ankle surgeon must master, and is presented in detail.

Traumatic foot and ankle injuries in the high-risk surgical patient are usually treated conservatively under the erroneous belief that this is the only means of maintaining the lower limb. However, the use of advanced percutaneous and minimum incision internal fixation and external fixation techniques, which respect regional vascular flow and provide ample stability, represent viable options in this patient population.

The use of autogenous bone graft and bone marrow aspirate for osseous healing is not new; however, the ability to harvest these products from the lower extremity has received relatively little attention and is discussed in this issue of *Clinics* in order to provide the readers with a safe, effective, and reproducible means of performing these useful techniques.

The topics discussed should allow the creative foot and ankle surgeon to expand their ability to provide high-risk surgical patients with a stable, plantigrade, and well-balanced foot capable of accepting the repeated stress of ambulation, rather than the proverbial "glass slipper," which repeatedly ulcerates or develops progressive deformity with use.

It is hoped that the readers of this issue of *Clinics of Podiatric Medicine and Surgery* will enjoy these articles and benefit from the surgical experience of the authors selected as much as I have.

Thomas S. Roukis, DPM, FACFAS
Chief, Limb Preservation Service
Director, Limb Preservation Complex Lower Extremity Surgery and
Research Fellowship
Vascular/Endovascular Surgery Service
Department of Surgery
Madigan Army Medical Center
9040-A Fitzsimmons Avenue, MCHJ-SV
Tacoma, WA 98431, USA

E-mail address: thomas.s.roukis@us.army.mil

ELSEVIER
SAUNDERS

Clin Podiatr Med Surg
25 (2008) 547–569

CLINICS IN
PODIATRIC
MEDICINE AND
SURGERY

Tenotomy and Tendon Transfer About the Forefoot, Midfoot and Hindfoot

Adam Landsman, DPM, PhD, FACFAS[a,b,*],
Emily Cook, DPM, AACFAS[a,b],
Jeremy Cook, DPM, AACFAS[a,b]

[a]Harvard Medical School, Boston, MA, USA
[b]Division of Podiatric Surgery, Department of Surgery, Beth Israel Deaconess
Medical Center, One Deaconess Road, Palmer-Baker Span 3, Boston, MA 02215, USA

Soft-tissue contractures about the foot and especially the forefoot are common deformities. These soft-tissue contractures create deformities that can be difficult if not impossible to accommodate without surgical intervention in the high-risk patient (ie, diabetes, peripheral neuropathy, immunosuppression, corticosteroid use, malnutrition, noncompliance) [1–8]. Although myriad techniques exist for soft-tissue rebalancing, including tendon lengthening and tendon transfer, a major limitation of any soft-tissu procedure is the inability to correct rigid deformities. Therefore, it is imperative to ascertain the degree of flexibility and range of motion present at the joint where the intended soft-tissue procedure is to be performed. Osseous procedures such as corrective osteotomies and realignment arthrodesis should be performed before tendon lengthening or transfer.

The authors present a detailed review of various tendon-lengthening and tendon- transfer procedures about the forefoot, midfoot, and hindfoot useful for the high-risk patient with a flexible deformity or following osseous surgery to realign the foot. A detailed review of surgical techniques to address soft-tissue ankle equinus [9] and techniques employed to balance partial foot amputations [10] are presented elsewhere in this issue.

* Corresponding author. Division of Podiatric Surgery, Department of Surgery, Beth Israel Deaconess Medical Center, Harvard Medical School, One Deaconess Road, Boston, MA 02215.
E-mail address: alandsma@bidmc.harvard.edu (A. Landsman).

Forefoot contractures

Forefoot contractures involve deformities about the toes and metatarsal–phalangeal joints that develop from intrinsic muscle wasting and biomechanical imbalances as is seen commonly in patients who have diabetic motor neuropathy. In combination with peripheral sensory and autonomic neuropathy, this may result in chronic ulceration at the distal tufts or dorsal aspects of flexed joints (Fig. 1) [1,2]. These deformities are exceedingly difficult to accommodate through conservative means and frequently deteriorate into a soft-tissue infection and contiguous-spread osteomyelitis (Fig. 2), ultimately resulting in digital amputation, ray resection, or partial foot amputation [8,11].

The underlying biomechanical etiology should be ascertained before procedure selection is made. It is important to appreciate that rigid deformities, or an abnormal metatarsal parabola will not respond as well to these soft-tissue techniques in isolation and should be approached with osseous procedures [8,12] alongside soft-tissue and tendon rebalancing as necessary. Other factors, including the patient's vascular status, extent of deformity, and location of any preulcerative lesion or formal ulceration will help choose the best procedure for each patient.

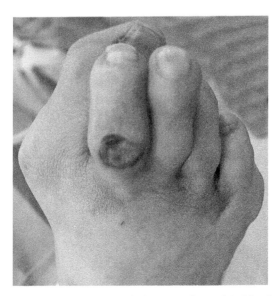

Fig. 1. Anterior–posterior clinical photograph demonstrating a global forefoot deformity with combined rigid and flexible toe deformities. Note the large hallux valgus deformity has resulted in dorsal contracture of the second toe, which has ulcerated at the proximal interphalangeal joint secondary to prolonged use of ill-fitting shoe gear with a narrow toe-box.

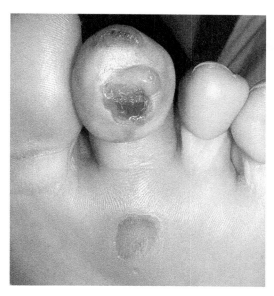

Fig. 2. En fass clinical photograph of an infected ulceration at the distal tip of the second toe associated with combined flexible and rigid toe contracture.

Percutaneous toe and metatarsal–phalangeal tenotomies

A percutaneous tenotomy of the long flexor tendon is frequently adequate for flexible contractures of the toes [13–18]. This is particularly evident in those patients who may present with distal tuft ulcerations (Fig. 3). If the patient has additional contracture at the metatarsal–phalangeal joint, another option is a long extensor tenotomy with or without metatarsal–phalangeal joint capsulotomy (Fig. 4) [17]. These percutaneous procedures are ideal for use in high-risk patients, because they can be performed under local anesthesia in a brief period of time with a high degree of success and without the use of a tourniquet.

The surgical technique begins with the patient positioned in a supine position on the operating room table. A tourniquet is not required, as the expected blood loss is minimal because of the limited soft-tissue dissection required for this procedure. Following regional infiltration of local anesthesia with or without monitored intravenous sedation, a 3 mm incision is drawn on the plantar aspect of the toe at the apex of the deformity, which is usually at the level of the proximal or distal interphalangeal joint. The incision is made perpendicular to the course of the tendon (ie, in line with the longitudinal axis of the toe) through the skin and carried down to the underlying flexor digitorum longus tendon. This tendon is transected under tension created by the surgeon's nondominant hand through simultaneous extension of the tip of the toe with the index finger and extension of the proximal interphalangeal joint with the thumb (see Fig. 3). Following

550 LANDSMAN et al

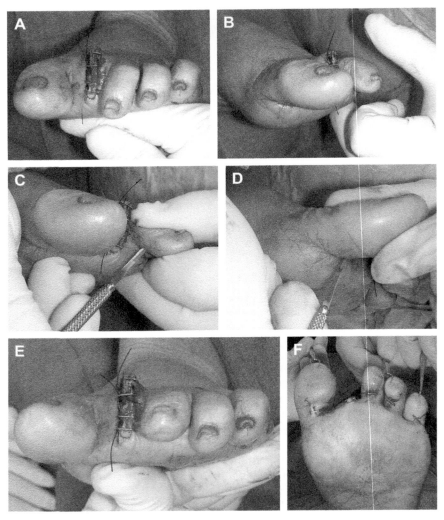

Fig. 3. Intraoperative en fass view of a patient following amputation of the second toe for osteomyelitis (*A*). The forefoot has been loaded in a dorsal direction to simulate weight bearing, and this reveals flexion contractures of the remaining toes at the interphalangeal joints and metatarsal–phalangeal joints. Intraoperative view demonstrating the proper approach to grasp the lesser toe (*B*) as described in the text as well as the incision location to perform percutaneous flexor tenotomy of the lesser toes (*C*) and hallux (*D*). Intraoperative en fass view following percutaneous flexor tenotomy of the hallux and third toe with the forefoot loaded in a dorsal direction (*E*). Note the resting extended position of the hallux and third toe compared with the adjacent toes and with *A*. Plantar view following percutaneous tenotomy of all remaining toes demonstrating the incision placement and closure technique as discussed in the text (*F*).

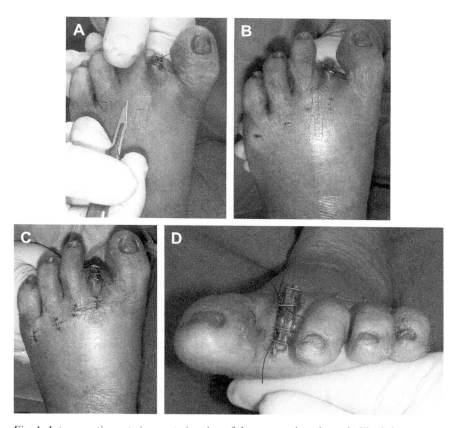

Fig. 4. Intraoperative anterior–posterior view of the same patient shown in Fig. 3 demonstrating plantarflexion of the third toe with slight distal traction along with a No. 11 blade, which is employed to transect the extensor tendon and perform a capsulotomy of the metatarsal–phalangeal joint as discussed in the text (*A*). Anterior–posterior view following completion of the extensor tenotomy and metatarsal–phalangeal joint capsulotomy as discussed in the text before (*B*) and following sin closure (*C*). En fass view with the forefoot loaded in a dorsal direction demonstrating the final result achieved following percutaneous flexor tenotomies and extensor tenotomy with metatarsal-phalangeal joint capsulotomy (*D*). Note the reduction of the deformities when compared with Fig. 3A.

transection of the flexor digitorum longus tendon, the toe is manipulated by first applying plantarly directed pressure to the proximal phalanx head with the surgeon's nondominant hand and then dorsally directed pressure on the distal phalanx. This releases any remaining flexor tendon fibers and disrupts the plantar plates to the proximal and distal interphalangeal joints (ie, phalangeal set procedure) [18], allowing full correction. If full correction is not achieved, the incision can be lengthened slightly to allow for insertion of a small curved hemostat, which is passed deep to the flexor digitorum longus and used to retract the tendon into the surgical field so that it can be transected under direct visualization. Once correction is achieved, the surgical site is closed with a single metallic staple or nylon suture.

If the toe contracture is corrected fully, but the metatarsal–phalangeal joint remains contracted, a percutaneous extensor tenotomy with or without capsulotomy can be performed. The toe is grasped in the surgeon's nondominant hand and simultaneously plantarflexed and distracted at the metatarsal–phalangeal joint. This places the extensor tendon and capsule under tension, and makes these structures more superficial. A No. 11 blade then is inserted through the skin overlying the metatarsal–phalangeal joint, and once through the skin, the tip of the blade is directed laterally and deepened a few millimeters. With the blade maintained at this level, the tip of the blade is rotated medially with care taken not to further incise the skin, and the extensor tendon is released. The toe is manipulated in plantarflexion at the metatarsal–phalangeal joint level, and the degree of correction is ascertained by loading the forefoot with dorsally directed pressure. If the release was complete, the toe will lie in a rectus position at the metatarsal–phalangeal joint and interphalangeal joints, assuming the flexor tenotomy was performed as described. If the correction at the metatarsal–phalangeal joint was not adequate, the blade can be reinserted into the incision and carried down to the metatarsal–phalangeal joint capsule, which is incised using the same technique for extensor tenotomy. Once correction appears adequate, the toe is plantarflexed at the metatarsal–phalangeal joint, and the skin is reapproximated with a single metallic staple (see Fig. 4).

Following completion of these procedures, a specialized dressing is applied and consists of gauze padding placed over the metatarsal–phalangeal joints dorsally, and at the plantar aspect of the toes, to maintain reduction of the toe deformities [17,18]. This is followed by application of a bulky, well-padded dressing from toes to knee [19]. The patient is allowed guarded full weight bearing in a postoperative shoe (Med-Surg, Darco International, Incorporated, Huntington, West Virginia) with a low-profile rocker sole and orthosis system (Peg-Assist, Darco International, Incorporated) that consists of layers of varying density and heat-moldable liners with a series of removable pegs that enhance shock absorption and off-loading, respectively. The initial surgical dressings are removed in 3 to 5 days, unless a wound is present that requires closer monitoring, and then every 7 to 10 days thereafter. Once fully healed, the patient gradually is returned toextradepth shoe gear with accommodative multidensity insoles for life [19].

Stephens [13], in a technique manuscript, described tenotomy of the flexor hallucis longus tendon at the base of the proximal phalanx to treat chronic plantar hallux ulcerations but provided no data. Laborde [16] evaluated 17 patients (17 feet) in whom he performed the same technique described by Stephens [13] and reported complete ulcer healing within 2 months without development of new toe deformities. Three ulcers recurred (18%) over time and were treated successfully with a repeat tenotomy that successfully healed the recurrent ulceration.

An abstract presented by Kirketerp-Moeller and colleagues [14] examined outcomes in patients who had neuropathic ulcerations following a toe flexor tenotomy. Each patient had a flexible contracted digit at either the proximal or distal interphalangeal joints. With a mean follow up of 3.1 months, 92% of the patients healed the ulcers in a median of 3 weeks after the procedure. Three patients did not heal, requiring a partial digital amputation in one case, while the remaining two cases needed a more extensive amputation. These failures were attributed to ischemia and gross infection [14]. Laborde [16] evaluated 11 patients (11 feet) in whom he performed the same technique described by Kirketerp-Moeller and colleagues [14] and reported complete ulcer healing within 2 months for all ulcerations without development of new toe deformities.

Although the literature is sparse regarding the use of percutaneous extensor and flexor tenotomy and metatarsal-phalangeal joint capsulotomy in high-risk patients, these techniques appear safe and effective at reducing flexible digital deformities in patients considered at high risk for toe ulceration, which can lead to amputation.

Extensor hallucis longus and flexor hallucis longus tendon transfers

The extensor hallucis longus transfer to the first metatarsal neck (ie, Jones tenosuspension) is indicated in the presence of a clawing of the hallux (ie, hallux malleus), along with a flexible plantarflexed first metatarsal. This procedure may be indicated in patients who have flexible deformity causing ulcerations plantar to the first metatarsal head or dorsally over the hallux interphalangeal joint because of contracture [20]. Consideration should be given to an adjunctive hallux interphalangeal joint arthrodesis to prevent progressive hallux contracture formation following this procedure [21]. Alternatively, a transfer of the flexor hallucis longus tendon to the base of the proximal phalanx of the hallux has been shown in a cadaver model to achieve similar correction at the metatarsal–phalangeal and interphalangeal joint levels but does not require arthrodesis of the hallux interphalangeal joint [20,22,23].

One cause of this constellation of symptoms is weakness of the tibialis anterior, resulting in plantarflexion of the forefoot [20,21]. Its antagonist, peroneus longus, overpowers the tibialis anterior in this situation and plantarflexes the first ray. Compensation by means of the extensor hallucis longus in this setting acts as a supplementary dorsiflexor of the ankle joint. With the prolonged activity of the extensor hallucis longus throughout the gait cycle, the first metatarsal–phalangeal joint can become fixed in a hyperextended position. Retrograde buckling occurs and further drives the first metatarsal head plantarly, resulting in an increased amount of force, which can lead to ulceration [20–23]. By transferring the extensor hallucis longus tendon to the first metatarsal neck, the deforming force acting upon the hallux instead is used to dorsiflex the first metatarsal and ankle.

Other options include peroneus longus tenotomy, lengthening, or transfer, as well as transfer of the flexor hallucis longus tendon described previously [20,21].

The extensor hallucis longus tendon transfer is performed with the patient positioned in a supine position on the operating room table. A tourniquet is not required, as the expected blood loss is minimal because of the limited soft-tissue dissection required for this procedure. One however, may be applied if indicated based on other concomitant procedures being performed after verifying appropriate vascular status. Following regional infiltration of local anesthesia with or without monitored intravenous sedation, a 5 cm linear incision is made along the medial border of the extensor hallucis longus tendon. The distal extent of the incision should be 1 cm distal to the hallux interphalangeal joint to allow for adequate dissection. Dissection is carried down to the extensor hallucis longus tendon deep to the subcutaneous adipose tissue. The extensor hallucis longus tendon is transected just proximal to the hallux interphalangeal joint and tagged with nonabsorbable suture. Traditionally, the extensor hallucis longus tendon has been transferred through a transverse drill hole from medial-to-lateral in the first metatarsal neck and sutured back onto itself. This method is very stable and has the advantage of increased bone-to-tendon surface contact. The disadvantages include the requirement of more extensive dissection particularly laterally and a greater degree of technical difficulty. For these reasons, the authors prefer to secure the extensor hallucis longus tendon transfer with the use of an absorbable interference screw, oriented dorsal-to-plantar, placed in the central aspect of the first metatarsal head. Although this technique is simpler to perform and requires less dissection when compared with the traditional method, it is essential that before insertion of the interference screw, proper tensioning of the tendon is achieved. Assessment of the metatarsal correction is analyzed, and excess tendon may be removed to achieve appropriate tension. Following completion of the tendon transfer, the hallux interphalangeal joint can be prepared for arthrodesis and fixated with an internal compression screw, one or two staples, or crossed Kirschner wires. The distal stump of the extensor hallucis longus tendon is tenodesed to the extensor hallucis brevis tendon to preserve some functional extension of the first metatarsal–phalangeal joint.

For a flexor hallucis longus transfer, the patient is positioned in an identical fashion; however, the incision placement is medially between the first metatarsal–phalangeal joint proximally and the hallux interphalangeal joint distally. Dissection is carried down to the underlying capsular structures, which are incised at the plantar aspect to access the flexor hallucis longus tendon, which is followed distally to its terminal insertion on the base of the distal phalanx of the hallux. Following transection, the flexor hallucis longus tendon either is passed through a plantar-to-dorsal drill hole and sutured to the extensor hallucis longus tendon or secured with the use of an interference screw as discussed previously.

When using either technique, the transferred tendons are secured to the surrounding tissues with use of heavy gauge nonabsorbable sutures, followed by capsular and periosteal tissue closure and skin reapproximation. A bulky, well-padded dressing then is applied from toes to knee, with or without supplemental use of a sugar tong plaster splint. The patient is immobilized until all skin sutures and staples are removed. Once fully healed, the patient gradually is returned to extradepth shoe gear with accommodative multidensity insoles for life [19].

A retrospective study of the extensor hallucis longus tendon transfer technique evaluated 28 feet (24 patients) with a mean follow-up of 5.5 years. Indications for the procedure were clawing of the hallux in 30% of patients, need to alleviate pressure plantar to the first metatarsal head in 55%, and a combination of both symptoms in 13%. Correction of the hallux claw toe was effective in 90% of cases; however, only 43% of patients noted resolution of plantar first metatarsal head pain. Three patients reported the pain had resolved initially but recurred within 18 months. This was particularly evident in those patients who had a less flexible deformity of the first metatarsal–phalangeal joint [24].

Several studies have evaluated the effectiveness of the flexor hallucis longus tendon transfer and compared this technique to the extensor hallucis tendon transfer for correction of hallux claw toe associated with a flexible plantarflexed first metatarsal [20,22,23]. Kadel and colleagues [20] retrospectively reviewed 22 feet (19 patients) that had flexor hallucis longus tendon transfer for correction of hallux claw toe with a mean follow-up of 5 months (range: 6 to 74 months). The authors noted radiographic improvement of the hallux interphalangeal joint and first metatarsal–phalangeal joint angles on lateral weight-bearing radiographs in all feet. Thirteen patients were fully satisfied, and six were somewhat satisfied with the overall result of the surgery. Four patients thought that their hallux limited the types of shoes they could wear, while 15 did not.

Steensma and colleagues [23] conducted a retrospective review of 6 patients with a mean follow-up of 24 plus or minus 15.2 months who had a flexor hallucis longus tendon transfer to the proximal phalanx of the great toe for hallux claw toe deformity. All deformities were corrected; pain was improved reliably at the plantar aspect of the first metatarsal head, and alignment was maintained at the time of final follow-up. All six patients treated for hallux claw deformity were satisfied with their outcomes. The authors concluded that the flexor hallucis longus transfer to the proximal phalanx appears to be a viable treatment option for hallux claw deformity in terms of deformity correction, pain relief, and patient satisfaction. These studies reported similar results between the extensor hallucis longus and flexor hallucis longus transfer procedures with the added benefit of not requiring arthrodesis of the hallux interphalangeal joint when transfer of the flexor hallucis longus tendon was performed [20,22,23].

Midfoot contractures

Patients undergoing a transmetatarsal (Fig. 5A) or midfoot level
(Fig. 5B) amputation must be evaluated properly to address tendon imbalances that create an equinus contracture of the ankle and varus contracture
of the residual foot for the reasons described elsewhere in this issue [9,10].
Soft-tissue equinus contracture is addressed through percutaneous tendo-
Achilles lengthening, open gastrocnemius recession, or endoscopic gastrocnemius recession [9]. Correction of the varus contracture of the residual foot
can be achieved with a peroneus brevis to peroneus longus transfer [10,25],
intramedullary screw fixation across the medial column joints of the foot
[10,26], or transfer of the tibialis anterior tendon to the lateral cuneiform
or cuboid [27,28]. Each of these procedures offsets the supinatory forces
across the midtarsal and subtalar joints and restores the residual partial
foot amputation to a plantigrade posture.

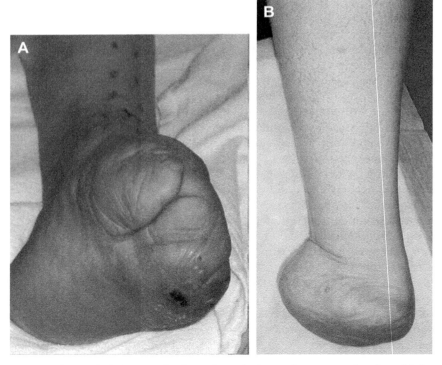

Fig. 5. En fass clinical photograph of a patient who has undergone a series of partial foot
amputations that have not been balanced appropriately, leading to an equinus–varus foot posture and associated plantar–lateral residual foot ulcerations (A). Clinical photograph of the medial aspect of the residual foot following midtarsal joint amputation performed without tendon
balancing (B). Note the severe equinus–varus foot posture.

With more proximal amputations, such as tarsal-metatarsal joint (ie, Lisfranc) and midtarsal joint (ie, Chopart) amputations, all anterior and lateral muscle groups have been released, leaving only posterior muscle group attachments. Without aggressive soft-tissue balancing, the foot will be left in equinus–varus posture creating distal–lateral residual foot amputation ulcerations. Careful isolation and transfer of tendons from the anterior and lateral compartments along with lengthening of the superficial and deep posterior compartments of the lower leg should be performed. As noted previously, soft-tissue equinus contracture is addressed through percutaneous tendo-Achilles lengthening, open gastrocnemius recession, or endoscopic gastrocnemius recession [9]. Varus contracture is addressed through transfer of the tibialis anterior to the medial cuneiform [28] and transfer of the peroneus brevis to the cuboid in tarsal–metatarsal amputations [10] and transfer of the tibialis anterior tendon to the neck of the talus [29] or through transfer of the peroneus longus to the tibialis anterior tendon under the neck of the talus to act as a stirrup that maintains the residual foot in rectus alignment.

Tibialis anterior tendon transfer

Regardless of amputation level, when considering transfer of the anterior tibial tendon, its power must be examined closely to determine if only part or if the entire tendon should be transferred. If its antagonistic muscle, peroneus longus, is left intact, it should be evaluated also. Once the tibialis anterior is transferred, the peroneus longus will gain mechanical advantage. If there is ulceration beneath the first metatarsal region because of a strong peroneus longus muscle, other alternative tendon transfers should be considered. At the conclusion of the tibialis anterior transfer, the toes also should be examined. When bringing the foot out of plantarflexion, hammertoe deformities may result because of remaining contracted long flexor tendons. If this occurs, flexor tenotomies can rectify this as described previously.

With the patient positioned on the operating room table in the supine position and a well-padded gel bolster placed under the ipsilateral buttock to control physiologic external rotation of the lower limb, the foot, ankle, lower leg, and thigh are prepped and draped in aseptic technique. A tourniquet is not necessary because of the limited soft-tissue dissection using well-placed incisions that respect the regional vascular structures. Three incisions will be required to perform either the split or complete tibialis anterior tendon transfer. Osseous landmarks first are drawn on the foot and lower leg, identifying the anterior tibial crest, ankle joint line, navicular tuberosity, medial cuneiform, first metatarsal base, lateral cuneiform, and cuboid. Especially for the lateral cuneiform or cuboid, a 25-gauge needle placed under fluoroscopy can be very helpful to avoid unnecessarily large incisions (Fig. 6). Preoperatively, the tibialis anterior tendon can be marked out by having the patient invert and dorsiflex his or her foot. In addition, a Doppler

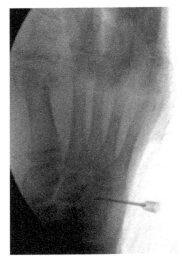

Fig. 6. Intraoperative image intensification anterior–posterior view demonstrating the use of a 25-gauge needle to isolate the cuboid, which is the intended tendon transfer location.

ultrasound probe is used preoperatively and postoperatively to confirm a patent anterior tibial and dorsalis pedis artery, especially if the patient has had a pedal bypass graft. In fact, the authors have observed a case in which a recent pedal bypass graft was occluded following overzealous tightening of the tibialis anterior tendon following transfer.

The first incision is placed directly over the insertion of the tibialis anterior tendon overlying the medial cuneiform. The second incision should be directly over the tibialis anterior tendon within the distal one third of the lower leg, just lateral to the anterior tibial crest; this is typically 7 to 8 cm proximal to the ankle joint. Finally, the third incision is centered directly over the target location of the tendon transfer, which is usually the lateral cuneiform or cuboid. Following isolation of the distal and proximal portions of the tibialis anterior tendon, the proximal section of the tendon is incised longitudinally, and umbilical tape is passed through this longitudinal split to equally divide the tendon into medial and lateral portions [30]. Long tendon-passing hemostats are passed from the distal incision into the proximal one, being careful to follow the course of the tibialis anterior tendon. This clamp then grasps the umbilical tape proximally. While maintaining tension on the tendon, the umbilical tape is pulled distally toward the tibialis anterior tendon insertion to divide the tendon into two halves. At this point, the lateral half is transected free as distally as possible, and retrieved into the proximal incision. If performing a complete tibialis anterior tendon transfer, the use of umbilical tape is not necessary. Attention then is directed to the third incision, directly over the target area for the transfer. This is frequently the lateral cuneiform or cuboid and previously has been marked and identified under intraoperative image intensification. The harvested tibialis anterior tendon should be kept moist while preparing this site. Dissection is carried down to the tendon target insertion site. If using a soft-tissue anchor, it may be inserted at this time, confirming the position and alignment under intraoperative image intensification. The long tendon passing hemostat then is tunneled from the distal lateral incision to the proximal lower leg incision, with care being taken to remain deep to the extensor retinaculum. This step is important to prevent bowstringing of the tendon. The long hemostat then grasps the tendon tag and pulls the tibialis anterior tendon from proximal to distal, deep to the extensor retinaculum. The foot then is held in the corrected position. If the entire tendon is being transferred, the foot usually is held in a more everted and dorsiflexed position. If a split tibialis anterior tendon transfer is performed, however, the foot is held in dorsiflexion with equal amounts of tension medially and laterally between the two tendon halves. The tendon then is anchored laterally into either the lateral cuneiform or cuboid. Although there are many acceptable methods for anchoring the tendon, the authors advocate the use of an interference screw [31]. This method requires less tendon length, and excellent tension can be achieved when the tendon is pulled alongside of the interference screw during anchoring [31].

One large study evaluated split tibialis anterior tendon transfer in 73 feet for equinus–varus deformities secondary to anoxic brain injury and cerebral vascular accident. Patients' autonomy significantly improved with a statistically significant increase in the ability to independently ambulate and wear normal shoes [32]. This transfer also is felt to be less predictable than others, however. The main concern with split transfers is obtaining balanced tension between the two halves [33]. More recent studies have indicated that the tibialis anterior becomes an evertor of the subtalar joint throughout its entire range of motion. If this is the desired effect, then this is an appropriate transfer. Otherwise, if only a small amount of eversion is desired, a less aggressive alternative should be chosen [34]. The optimal transfer site also always is not determined easily. For instance, a study by Hui and colleagues [35] found that to primarily increase dorsiflexion and minimize pronatory moments, transfer into the third or fourth metatarsals was recommended.

Peroneus longus to peroneus brevis tendon transfer

Various circumstances can lead to weakness of the pronators of the foot. Neurologic disorders such as Charcot-Marie-Tooth are one such example, but chronic tears and even the consequences of a lateral ankle stabilization procedure can diminish this action also [36]. Regardless of the cause, this can result in overload of the lateral column and increase the risk of ulceration. Although a weak evertor by comparison, a transfer of the peroneus longus to the peroneus brevis can be effective in reestablishing pronation about the midtarsal joint. In addition, this procedure can be used to alleviate force under the first metatarsophalangeal joint.

With the patient positioned on the operating room table in the supine position and a well-padded gel bolster placed under the ipsilateral buttock to control physiologic external rotation of the lower limb, or with the patient in a lateral decubitus position, the foot, ankle, lower leg, and thigh are prepared and draped in aseptic technique. A tourniquet is not necessary because of the limited soft-tissue dissection using well-placed incisions that respect the regional vascular structures. It may be employed, however, if indicated based on other surgical procedures and verification of the patient's vascular status as adequate. An approximately 4 to 5 cm linear incision is made over the course of the peroneal tendons as previously described [10,25] and carried down to the level of the peroneal retinaculum. With the foot in neutral position, the peroneus longus tendon is transected approximately 1 cm proximal to its entrance at the cuboid notch and tagged with nonabsorbable suture. Attention is directed to the peroneus brevis tendon 0.5 to 1 cm proximal to its insertion on the fifth metatarsal base. The tendon is marked with electrocautery at two or three locations along its length for the reasons previously described [10,25], followed by full-thickness tenotomy incisions. The peroneus longus tendon then is weaved through the peroneus brevis, starting at the proximal tenotomy site and continued distally until the weave is completed. With the foot maintained in neutral position, the transferred peroneus longus tendon then is sutured to the peroneus brevis throughout its length. Unless this procedure was performed to alleviate pressures plantar to the first metatarsal head, the distal peroneus longus tendon stump should be attached to the cuboid to limit the potential for a dorsally unstable first metatarsal. This can be achieved by direct suturing to the cuboid periosteum or with the use of a soft-tissue anchor. Regardless of the method of attachment, by carefully tensioning the peroneus longus tendon stump, the first metatarsal is maintained in a static and supported position.

Hamilton and colleagues [37] combined this procedure with a gastrocnemius recession and lesser metatarsal head resections in 12 feet for the treatment of forefoot ulceration. The role of the peroneus longus transfer was to reduce the risk of transfer lesion formation plantar to the intact first metatarsal head. With a mean follow-up of 14.1 months, 100% of the patients were free of transfer lesions and recurrent ulceration [37].

Hindfoot contractures

Hindfoot contractures include equinus contracture, which is described elsewhere in this issue [9]; drop foot; and calcaneal deformities, which will be described here. Most surgical techniques described to correct the drop foot deformity have been applied to correct the absence of active dorsiflexion as a result of the loss of lower leg anterior compartment muscle function, and to correct the cavus–varus deformities caused by the combined contracture of the deep posterior and lateral lower leg musculature. The mainstay of surgical correction involving tendon transfers has revolved around the transmembranous or circum–tibial transfer of the tibialis posterior tendon with or without concomitant transfer of the flexor hallucis longus or peroneus longus tendons to the dorsum of the foot [38–41]. One concern with this approach is the development of dorsal–lateral peri-talar subluxation following transfer of the tibialis posterior tendon [42]. Additionally, some patients with drop foot deformity such as those following a cerebral vascular accident [43] or following bariatric surgery [44] are considered high-risk for a major tendon transfer such as a tibialis posterior transfer and the associated protracted recovery, which necessitates musculotendinous rehabilitation and training. An alternative approach is a tenodesis of the tibialis anterior to the tibia [45,46] to form a tenosuspension intended to maintain the foot in neutral position so that bracing can be employed rather than attempting to create dynamic dorsiflexion. This approach is much more simplistic and requires little dissection to perform properly. Regardless of what surgical procedure is performed to correct the drop foot deformity, correction of the associated soft-tissue ankle equinus should be performed before correcting the drop foot deformity, as described elsewhere in this issue [9].

Tibialis anterior tenosuspension

Tibialis anterior tenosuspension does not allow for the tibialis anterior to provide active dorsiflexion of the foot. It produces a sound suspension tenodesis, however, which corrects the foot slap component of the drop foot deformity and does allow for some active dorsiflexion when the peroneus tertius is functioning because the enhanced mechanical advantage created. This technique is simpler to perform than tendon transfers that transfer the distal attachment of the tendon to a new location in the foot itself or with tendon-weaving techniques. Additionally, because the distal insertion site is left intact, tibialis anterior tenosuspension is more secure than other transfer techniques.

With the patient positioned on the operating room table in the supine position and a well-padded gel bolster placed under the ipsilateral buttock to control physiologic external rotation of the lower limb, the foot, ankle, lower leg, and thigh are prepared and draped in an aseptic manner. A tourniquet is not necessary because of the limited soft-tissue dissection using well-placed incisions that respect the regional vascular structures. It may be employed, however, if indicated based on other surgical procedures and verification of the patient's vascular status as adequate. Under intravenous sedation and popliteal block anesthesia, a 3 cm long incision is placed approximately 10cm proximal to the medial malleolus and directly medial to the tibialis anterior tendon. Following dissection through the subcutaneous tissues, the tibialis anterior tendon sheath is identified and incised linearly to expose the underlying tendon, which is retracted from the wound and transected at the proximal extent of the incision near the musculotendinous junction. The periosteum overlying the medial crest of the distal tibia then is roughened with a rotary burr to aide in tenodesis. The tibialis anterior tendon is pulled proximally until the foot is in the desired plantigrade position and then secured to the underlying tibia through the use of one or two 4 mm solid cancellous screws and two small spiked washers (Fig. 7). The strength of the tenosuspension is tested and the final resting foot posture examined for proper alignment before irrigation, deep subcutaneous tissue closure, and skin reapproximation. A short-leg weight-bearing cast then is applied for 3 weeks, followed by a removable short-leg walking boot for 3 weeks, during which the patient receives physical therapy for strengthening of the remaining lower leg musculature. The patient then is transitioned into an ankle–foot orthosis and extradepth shoe gear for life.

Tibialis posterior tendon transfer

Tibialis posterior tendon transfer through the interosseous membrane originally was presented for treating flaccid paralytic disorders such as

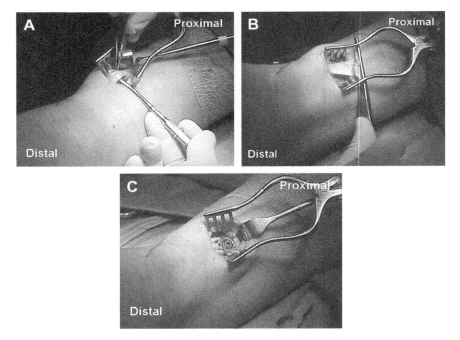

Fig. 7. Intraoperative view of the lower leg demonstrating identification of the tibialis anterior tendon (*A*), which is transected and pulled proximally until the foot resides in slight dorsiflexion at the ankle (*B*). The tendon then is secured to the underlying prepared medial aspect of the tibia with the use of a screw and spiked washer (*C*).

leprosy and poliomyelitis [38,39]. Later, its indications widened to include entities such as peroneal nerve palsy [40] and spastic disorders like cerebral palsy [41].

With the patient positioned on the operating room table in the supine position and a well-padded gel bolster placed under the ipsilateral buttock to control physiologic external rotation of the lower limb, the foot, ankle, lower leg, and thigh are prepared and draped in an aseptic manner. A tourniquet is not necessary because of the limited soft-tissue dissection using well-placed incisions that respect the regional vascular structures. It may be employed, however, if indicated based on other surgical procedures and verification of the patient's vascular status as adequate. Under intravenous sedation and popliteal block anesthesia, four incisions are required for this procedure, two medial and two anterior–dorsal, with each surface having a foot and lower leg incision. The tibialis posterior tendon is harvested through a 3 to 4 cm linear incision parallel to its course between the medial malleolus and dorsal aspect of the navicular. A frequently encountered obstacle is failure to obtain adequate tendon length, which will hamper efforts later in the procedure. To avoid this, the authors recommend dissecting the tendon as distally as possible through this incision and also including a small portion of the navicular tuberosity along with the tendon harvest, which maintains osseous tendon integrity useful for later insertion into an osseous tunnel in the lateral midfoot. The distal end of the tibialis posterior tendon is tagged with heavy-gauge nonabsorbable suture. The next incision is at the medial surface of the lower leg, where an incision in line with the posterior–medial border of the tibia is made approximately 8 to 10 cm proximal to the distal tip of the medial malleolus. At this level, it is common to visualize the flexor digitorum longus tendon that lies superficial to the tibialis posterior tendon. Once the tibialis posterior tendon is identified proximally, tension is applied to withdraw the entire tendon through the incision. A third incision then is made approximately 3 to 4 cm distal to the second incision on the anterior surface of the lower leg. This incision should be larger than the previous incisions, at approximately 4 to 6 cm, and also in line with the long axis of the tibia. The deep fascia should be incised lateral to the tibialis anterior tendon, which should be retracted laterally. This technique minimizes the risk of violating the adjacent neurovascular bundle. These structures should be visualized carefully before creating the interosseous membrane window, which involves resection of a long and wide strip to allow easy passage of the tibialis posterior muscle belly to limit tethering. The tibialis posterior tendon then is passed from posterior-to-anterior through the window within the interosseous membrane. The final incision is made over the intermediate cuneiform approximately 2 to 3 cm in length. A long clamp is placed through this incision deep to the extensor retinaculum toward the anterior lower leg incision, where the tibialis posterior tendon is grasped and pulled distally through the lateral foot incision. Traditionally, an osseous tunnel was described as being passed through the intermediate cuneiform and emerging out the plantar surface. Refinement of bone anchor technology such as the use of an interference screw has made this portion of the procedure significantly simpler, especially if a segment of the navicular was included with the original harvest, because this allows for bone-on-bone healing rather than tendon-on-bone, which takes significantly longer to incorporate [47]. Regardless of fixation technique, the final position of the foot is critical to patient outcome. During the tendon- anchoring phase, the foot should be dorsiflexed slightly at the ankle and slightly everted. Numerous modifications to the tibialis posterior tendon transfer have been advocated, but none proven superior [48–51]. Careful protection in a short-leg cast with progression to a removable boot over a 6 to 8 weeks should be performed, followed by transition into extradepth shoe gear with or without the use of a dorsiflexion assist ankle–foot orthosis for life. Aggressive physical therapy is required to retrain the tibialis posterior muscle to function out of phase, which is difficult to achieve in elderly, high-risk patients who have neuropathy.

Several studies have examined this procedure in the high-risk foot and supported its utility. A study by Gunn and Molesworth [39] reported an 87.5% satisfactory outcome in 56 feet with flaccid drop foot deformities. In a similar population, Pinzur and colleagues [40] noted 100% correction of the deformities without the need for subsequent bracing. Electromyography following this procedure confirmed dorsiflexory activity during gait in this study also [40]. Spastic conditions have proven to be less successful with this procedure. Root and colleagues [41] examined this procedure for treating spastic equinus–varus deformity in 57 patients who had cerebral palsy. With a mean follow-up of 9.3 years, 28% of patients had a poor outcome, with only 38% having a good outcome [41].

Flexor hallucis longus and peroneus brevis to Achilles tendon transfers

A commonly cited problem in the high-risk foot is that of iatrogenic calcaneal gait secondary to overlengthening or frank rupture of the Achilles tendon during surgical lengthening [9,52–55]. Although sparsely reported, this is a devastating iatrogenic injury that can result in a plantar-central heel ulceration and contiguous spread osteomyelitis of the calcaneus, which is exceedingly difficult to treat in the high-risk patient such as an obese, diabetic patient who has dense peripheral neuropathy. Besides tibial talus calcaneal arthrodesis, functional restoration of plantarflexion power can be attempted through the use of flexor hallucis longus [56–59] or peroneus brevis tendon transfers [59,60] to the distal insertion of the Achilles tendon or body of the calcaneus.

Advantages of the flexor hallucis longus tendon transfer include ease of harvest and a low-lying muscle belly that can be used for enhanced perfusion of the Achilles tendon [56–59]. Additionally, the muscle strength of the flexor hallucis longus is superior to the peroneus brevis [60,61]. According to a study performed by Silver and colleagues [61], the flexor hallucis longus contributes 3.6% to the effort of flexion as compared with the 2.6% of the peroneus brevis. This is minimal relative to the contribution of the gastrocnemius–soleus complex, which is 49.1%. With this structure compromised, however, additional plantarflexion power is necessary.

With either technique, the patient is positioned on the operating room table in the prone position with all osseous prominences appropriately padded, and the foot, ankle, lower leg, and thigh are prepared and draped using an aseptic technique. A tourniquet usually is employed to ease dissection but is not mandatory. Under general, spinal, or popliteal block anesthesia with intravenous sedation, the procedures may be performed through single or double incisions. If moderate lengths of the flexor hallucis longus or peroneus brevis tendons are required, a two-incision approach will give the surgeon more length to work with. With the use of interference screws and newer bone anchors, less tendon length is needed allowing flexor hallucis longus tendon harvest through a single posterior incision [59,62]. A disadvantage of the single-incision approach is that it will not be possible to tenodese the distal end of the transected flexor hallucis longus tendon into the flexor digitorum longus tendon, which may create weakness of hallux flexion during ambulation. Likewise, transfer of the transected peroneus brevis into the peroneus longus is difficult to perform and can alter midfoot function, leading to deformity.

When using the two-incision approach, an approximately 6 to 8 cm long linear incision is made over the midline of the Achilles tendon, although this incision can be biased medially for harvest of the flexor hallucis longus tendon and lateral for harvest of the peroneus brevis tendon. Dissection is carried down to the Achilles tendon paratenon, which is incised and protected for later closure. Following complete debridement of the Achilles tendon to remove all diseased components, the distal stump of the Achilles tendon should be inspected, and if attached securely, the tendon transfer can be weaved through it. Alternatively, the body of the calcaneus can be exposed just anterior to the Achilles tendon insertion for transfer of the tendon. The flexor hallucis longus tendon is identified coursing from lateral-to-medial deep to the Achilles tendon, along with its low-lying muscle belly. After incising the deep fascia, tension should be placed on the flexor hallucis longus tendon to verify that the hallux plantarflexes at the interphalangeal joint so as to avoid iatrogenic injury to adjacent neurovascular and tendinous structures. A flexible metallic probe then is passed down the sheath of the flexor hallucis longus to the level of the midfoot, and at this location, a 1 to 2 cm incision is placed and dissected down through the plantar fascia of the flexor hallucis longus tendon at the level where it interconnects with the flexor digitorum longus tendon (ie, Master knot of Henry) [63]. The flexor hallucis longus tendon is transected, with care taken not to injure the medial plantar nerve and artery [64,65], and the stump is secured to the flexor digitorum longus if possible to limit the potential for development of a hallux claw toe. The flexor hallucis longus tendon then is retrieved through the proximal incision. With the Achilles tendon site adequately prepared, the flexor hallucis longus muscle belly is mobilized to allow apposition with the proximal and distal segments of the Achilles tendon to afford vascularity and aide in repair. Delicate dissection off the tibia, fibula, and interosseous membrane is necessary to mobilize the flexor hallucis longus muscle belly distally and permit direct contact with the Achilles tendon. The final step of this procedure requires attachment of the flexor hallucis longus tendon, either through the intact insertion of the Achilles tendon through the use of sharp tendon-passing forceps, or into the body of the calcaneus with the use of soft-tissue anchors or inference screws as described previously [62]. The soft-tissue anchor or interference screw should be inserted with the ankle in slight plantarflexion and should be placed medial to the calcaneal midline to afford a supinatory force with contraction during gait. The flexor hallucis longus muscle belly then is sutured t directly o the Achilles tendon with nonabsorbable sutures. For peroneus brevis tendon transfer, a similar approach is used as was described for the flexor hallucis longus tendon transfer.

Regardless of which procedure is employed, the patient initially is placed into a sugar tong plaster splint, which is converted to a short-leg nonweight-bearing cast with the foot held in slight plantarflexion for approximately 6 to 8 weeks. This is followed by a weight-bearing short-leg cast with the foot held in neutral position for an additional 4 to 6 weeks with gradual return to an ankle–foot orthosis with dorsiflexion block and extradepth shoe gear for life.

There is a paucity of literature discussing the use of either flexor hallucis longus or peroneus brevis tendon transfers to restore plantarflexion power following iatrogenic overlengthening or rupture of the Achilles tendon following surgical lengthening. Chilvers and colleagues [55] described the use of flexor hallucis longus tendon transfer similar to that described here in two patients of a series of nine who had iatrogenic overlengthening of the Achilles tendon associated with heel ulceration. Their data reveal that three of the nine did not heal (33%); two healed with the use of a dorsiflexion stop ankle–foot orthosis, and one required a transtibial amputation. It should be understood that although flexor hallucis longus and peroneus brevis tendon transfers are options to restore plantarflexion power and divert plantar pressure from the heel pad, tendo-Achilles lengthening should be performed in a controlled fashion by experienced surgeons, or alternate techniques that involve gastrocnemius recession should be considered to avoid iatrogenic overlengthening or frank rupture as described elsewhere in this issue [9].

Summary

The authors present a detailed review of the most common tendon lengthening and transfer surgical procedures about the forefoot, midfoot, and hindfoot. These soft-tissue procedures are rarely performed in isolation and a detailed knowledge of additional soft-tissue and osseous surgical principles are mandatory. Tendon lengthening and transfer procedures about the forefoot, midfoot, and hindfoot represent an extremely powerful series of percutaneous or minimally invasive techniques that are capable of restoring form and function, and are useful when treating the high-risk patient.

References

[1] Frykberg RG. Diabetic foot ulcers: current concepts. J Foot Ankle Surg 1998;37(5):440–6.

[2] Isakov E, Budoragin N, Shenhav S, et al. Anatomic sites of foot lesions resulting in amputation among diabetics and nondiabetics. Am J Phys Med Rehabil 1995;74(2):130–3.

[3] Margolis DJ, Kantor J, Santanna J, et al. Risk factors for delayed healing of neuropathic diabetic foot ulcers: a pooled analysis. Arch Dermatol 2000;136(12):1531–5.

[4] Delbridge L, Perry P, Marr S, et al. Limited joint mobility in the diabetic foot: relationship to neuropathic ulceration. Diabet Med 1988;5(4):333–7.

[5] Mueller MJ, Diamond JE, Delitto A, et al. Insensitivity, limited joint mobility, and plantar ulcers in patients with diabetes mellitus. Phys Ther 1989;69(6):453–9.

[6] Fernando DJ, Masson EA, Veves A, et al. Relationship of limited joint mobility to abnormal foot pressures and diabetic foot ulceration. Diabetes Care 1991;14(1):8–11.

[7] Crisp AJ, Heathcote JG. Connective tissue abnormalities in diabetes mellitus. J R Coll Physicians Lond 1984;18(2):132–41.

[8] Sayner LR, Rosenblum BI, Giurini JM. Elective surgery of the diabetic foot. Clin Podiatr Med Surg 2003;20(4):783–92.

[9] Schweinberger MH, Roukis TS. Surgical correction of soft-tissue ankle equinus contracture. Clin Podiatr Med Surg 2008;25(4):571–85.

[10] Schweinberger MH, Roukis TS. Soft-tissue and osseous techniques to balance forefoot and midfoot amputations. Clin Podiatr Med Surg 2008;25(4):623–39.

[11] Öznur A, Roukis TS. Minimum incision ray resection. Clin Podiatr Med Surg 2008; 25(4):609–22.

[12] Roukis TS, Schade VL. Minimum incision metatarsal osteotomies. Clin Podiatr Med Surg 2008;25(4):587–607.

[13] Stephens HM. Technique tip: the diabetic plantar hallux ulcer: a curative soft-tissue procedure. Foot Ankle Int 2000;21(4):954–5.

[14] Kirketerp-Moeller K, Vestergaard ME, Holstein P. Flexor tenotomy in the management of ulcers of the toes of the diabetic foot. Abstract presented at the Diabetic Foot Study Group Scientific Meeting. Elsinore, Denmark, September 10–13, 2006.

[15] Lountzis N, Parenti J, Cush G, et al. Percutaneous flexor tenotomy: office procedure for diabetic toe ulcerations. Wounds 2007;19(3):64–8.

[16] Laborde JM. Neuropathic toe ulcers treated with toe flexor tenotomies. Foot Ankle Int 2007; 28(11):1160–4.

[17] Roven MD. Tenotomy, tenectomy, and capsulotomy for the lesser toes. Clin Podiatry 1985; 2(3):471–5.

[18] Roven MD. Phalangeal set. Clin Podiatry 1985;2(3):483–9.

[19] Andersen CA, Roukis TS. The diabetic foot. Surg Clin North Am 2007;87(5):1149–77.

[20] Kadel NJ, Donaldson-Fletcher EA, Hansen ST, et al. Alternative to the modified Jones procedure: outcomes of the flexor hallucis longus (FHL) tendon transfer procedure for correction of clawed hallux. Foot Ankle Int 2005;26(12):1021–6.

[21] Miller SJ, Groves MJ IV. Principles of muscle–tendon surgery and tendon transfers. In: Banks AS, Downey MS, Martin DE, et al, editors. McGlamry's Comprehensive textbook of foot and ankle surgery, 3rd edition, vol. 2. Philadelphia: Lippincott Williams & Wilkins; 2001. p. 1523–66.

[22] Elias FN, Yuen TJ, Olson SL, et al. Correction of clawed hallux deformity: comparison of the Jones procedure and FHL transfer in a cadaver model. Foot Ankle Int 2007;28(3):369–76.

[23] Steensma MR, Jabara M, Anderson JG, et al. Flexor hallucis longus tendon transfer for hallux claw toe deformity and vertical instability of the metatarsophalangeal joint. Foot Ankle Int 2006;27(9):689–92.

[24] Tynan MC, Klenerman L. The modified Robert Jones tendon transfer in cases of pes cavus and clawed hallux. Foot Ankle Int 1994;15(2):68–71.

[25] Schweinberger MH, Roukis TS. Balancing of the transmetatarsal amputation with peroneus brevis to peroneus longus tendon transfer. J Foot Ankle Surg 2007;46(6):510–4.

[26] Schweinberger MH, Roukis TS. Intramedullary screw fixation for balancing of the dysvascular foot following transmetatarsal amputation. J Foot Ankle Surg 2008;47.

[27] Clark G, Lui E, Cook K. Tendon balancing in pedal amputations. Clin Podiatr Med Surg 2005;22:447–67.

[28] Turan I. Tarsometatarsal amputation and tibialis anterior tendon transposition to cuneiform I. J Foot Surg 1985;24(2):113–5.

[29] Reyzelman AM, Hadi S, Armstrong DG. Limb salvage with Chopart's amputation and tendon balancing. J Am Podiatr Med Assoc 1999;89(2):100–3.

[30] Johnson CH. Tendon Transfers. In: Chang TJ, editor. Master techniques in podiatric surgery: the foot and ankle. Philadelphia: Lippincott Williams & Wilkins; 2005. p. 250–3.

[31] Fuller DA, McCarthy JJ, Keenan MA. The use of the absorbable interference screw for a split anterior tibial tendon (SPLATT) transfer procedure. Orthopedics 2004;27(4):372–4.

[32] Vogt JC. Split anterior tibial transfer for spastic equinovarus foot deformity: retrospective study of 73 operated feet. J Foot Ankle Surg 1998;37(1):2–7.

[33] Piazza SJ, Adamson RL, Sanders JO, et al. Changes in muscle moment arms following split tendon transfer of tibialis anterior and tibialis posterior. Gait Posture 2001;14(3):271–8.

[34] Piazza SJ, Adamson RL, Moran MF, et al. Effects of tensioning errors in split transfers of tibialis anterior and posterior tendons. J Bone Joint Surg Am 2003;85-A(5):858–65.

[35] Hui JH, Goh JC, Lee EH. Biomechanical study of tibialis anterior tendon transfer. Clin Orthop Relat Res 1998;349:249–55.

[36] Coughlin J. Disorders of tendons. In: Hurley R, editor. Surgery of the foot and ankle. 7th edition, vol. 2. St. Louis, Mosby; 1999. p. 786–861.

[37] Hamilton GA, Ford LA, Perez H, et al. Salvage of the neuropathic foot by using bone resection and tendon balancing: a retrospective review of 10 patients. J Foot Ankle Surg 2005;44: 37–44.

[38] Watkins MB, James JB, Ryder CT Jr, et al. Transplantation of the posterior tibial tendon. J Bone Joint Surg Am 1954;36(6):1181–9.

[39] Gunn DR, Molesworth BD. The use of tibialis anterior as a dorsiflexor. J Bone Joint Surg Br 1957;39(4):674–8.

[40] Pinzur MS, Kett N, Trilla M. Combined anteroposterior tibial tendon transfer in posttraumatic peroneal palsy. Foot Ankle 1988;8(5):271–5.

[41] Root L, Miller SR, Kirz P. Posterior tibial–tendon transfer in patients with cerebral palsy. J Bone Joint Surg Am 1987;69(8):1133–9.

[42] Vertullo CJ, Nunley JA. Acquired flatfoot deformity following posterior tibial tendon transfer for peroneal nerve injury. J Bone Joint Surg Am 2002;84(7):1214–7.

[43] Tsur A. Common peroneal neuropathy in patients after first-time stroke. Isr Med Assoc J 2007;9(12):866–9.

[44] Weyns FJ, Beckers F, Vanormelingen L, et al. Foot drop as a complication of weight loss after bariatric surgery: is it preventable? Obes Surg 2007;17(9):1209–12.

[45] Roukis TS, Landsman AS, Patel KE, et al. A simple technique for correcting footdrop: suspension tenodesis of the tibialis anterior tendon to the distal tibia. J Am Podiatr Med Assoc 2005;95(2):154–6.

[46] Turner JW, Cooper RR. Anterior transfer of the tibialis posterior through the interosseous membrane. Clin Orthop 1972;83:241–4.

[47] Buckwalter JA, Grodzinsky AJ. Loading of healing bone, fibrous tissue, and muscle: implications for orthopaedic practice. J Am Acad Orthop Surg 1999;7(5):291–9.

[48] Rodriguez RP. The Bridle procedure in the treatment of paralysis of the foot. Foot Ankle 1992;13:63–9.

[49] Prahinski JR, McHale KA, Temple HT, et al. Bridle transfer for paresis of the anterior and lateral compartment musculature. Foot Ankle Int 1996;17:615–9.

[50] Wagenaar FC, Lowerens JW. Posterior tibial tendon transfer: results of fixation to the dorsiflexors proximal to the ankle joint. Foot Ankle Int 2007;28(11):1128–42.

[51] Wagenaar FC, Lowerens JW. Technique tip: handling of the soft tissues of the anterior compartment in posterior tibial tendon transfer to the dorsiflexors proximal to the ankle joint. Foot Ankle Int 2007;28(11):1204–6.

[52] Mueller MJ, Sinacore DR, Hastings MK, et al. Effect of Achilles tendon lengthening on neuropathic plantar ulcers: a randomized clinical trial. J Bone Joint Surg Am 2003;85(8): 1436–45.

[53] Nishimoto GS, Attinger CE, Cooper PS. Lengthening the Achilles tendon for the treatment of diabetic plantar forefoot ulceration. Surg Clin North Am 2003;83(3):707–26.

[54] Holstein P, Lohmann M, Bitsch M, et al. Achilles tendon lengthening, the panacea for plantar forefoot ulceration? Diabetes Metab Res Rev 2004;20(Suppl 1):S37–40.

[55] Chilvers M, Malicky ES, Anderson JG, et al. Heel overload associated with heel cord insufficiency. Foot Ankle Int 2007;28(6):687–9.

[56] Wapner KL, Pavlock GS, Hecht PJ, et al. Repair of chronic Achilles tendon rupture with flexor hallucis longus tendon transfer. Foot Ankle 1993;14(8):443–9.

[57] Wong M, Ng S. Modified flexor hallucis longus transfer for Achilles insertional rupture in elderly patients. Clin Orthop 2005;431:201–6.

[58] Martin RL, Manning CM, Carcia CR, et al. An outcome study of chronic Achilles tendinosis after excision of the Achilles tendon and flexor hallucis longus tendon transfer. Foot Ankle Int 2005;26(9):691–7.

[59] Maffulli N, Ajis A, Longo UG, et al. Chronic rupture of tendo Achilles. Foot Ankle Clin 2007;12(4):583–96.

[60] Sebastian H, Datta B, Maffulli N, et al. Mechanical properties of reconstructed Achilles tendon with transfer of peroneus brevis or flexor hallucis longus tendon. J Foot Ankle Surg 2007;46(6):424–8.

[61] Silver RL, De La Garza J, Rang M. The myth of muscle balance: a study of relative muscle strengths and excursions of normal muscles about the foot and ankle. J Bone Joint Surg Br 1985;67(3):432–7.

[62] DeCarbo WT, Hyer CF. Interference screw fixation for flexor hallucis longus tendon transfer for chronic Achilles tendonopathy. J Foot Ankle Surg 2008;47(1):69–72.

[63] Panchbhavi VK, Trevino SG. Technique tip: minimally invasive technique for harvesting long flexor tendons of the foot. Foot Ankle Int 2007;28(2):269–71.

[64] Herbst SA, Miller SD. Transection of the medial plantar nerve and hallux cock-up deformity after flexor hallucis longus tendon transfer for Achilles tendinitis: case report. Foot Ankle Int 2006;27(8):639–41.

[65] Mulier T, Rummens E, Dereymaeker G. Risk of neurovascular injuries in flexor hallucis longus tendon transfers: an anatomic cadaver study. Foot Ankle Int 2007;28(8):910–5.

ELSEVIER
SAUNDERS

Clin Podiatr Med Surg
25 (2008) 571–585

CLINICS IN
PODIATRIC
MEDICINE AND
SURGERY

Surgical Correction of Soft-Tissue Ankle Equinus Contracture

Monica H. Schweinberger, DPM, AACFAS,
Thomas S. Roukis, DPM, FACFAS*

*Limb Preservation Service, Vascular/Endovascular Surgery Service, Department of Surgery,
Madigan Army Medical Center, 9040-A Fitzsimmons Avenue, MCHJ-SV,
Tacoma, WA 98431, USA*

Soft-tissue ankle equinus contracture is a limitation of dorsiflexion motion at the ankle joint and has been identified as a contributing factor in neuropathic ulceration and multiple foot deformities ranging from hallux valgus to Charcot neuro-osteoarthropathy [1–8]. Despite numerous publications on the equinus deformity, there remains disagreement as to what constitutes limited dorsiflexion at the ankle joint. With the knee extended, the reported normal range of ankle joint dorsiflexion in the literature varies from 3° to 15° [9–13], and with the knee flexed to 90°, the normal range has been reported from 10° to 20° or greater [10–12].

The Silfverskiold test (Fig. 1) has been used to differentiate between an isolated gastrocnemius equinus and a gastrocnemius–soleus equinus. Flexion of the knee will increase ankle joint range of motion in the case of an isolated gastrocnemius equinus, as it creates laxity in the gastrocnemius muscle, which originates from the posterior aspect of the femoral condyles, thereby crossing both the knee and the ankle joints [13]. When considering surgical correction of equinus, determination of whether to perform an open gastrocnemius recession (OGR) or endoscopic gastrocnemius recession (EGR), which only addresses the gastrocnemius muscle, or an Achilles tendon lengthening, which lengthens the combined tendon of the gastrocnemius and soleus muscles, traditionally has been based on the Silfverskiold test [1,14], assuming an osseous talotibial exostosis has

The opinions or assertions contained herein are the private views of the authors and are not to be construed as official or reflecting the views of the Department of the Army or the Department of Defense.

* Corresponding author.

E-mail address: thomas.s.roukis@us.army.mil (T.S. Roukis).

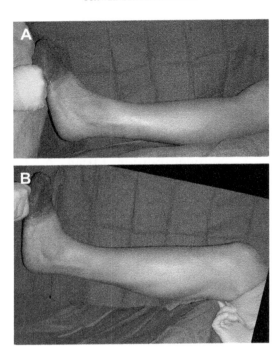

Fig. 1. Demonstration of the Silfverskiold test. With the knee extended, the rear foot is locked in varus, while the foot is dorsiflexed on the leg and the angle between the glabrous junction (where the dorsal and plantar skin meet) at the lateral foot and the longitudinal bisection of the fibula are measured (*A*). With the knee flexed at 90°, the foot is positioned as in *A* and dorsiflexed on the leg with the range of motion again measured in an identical manner (*B*). If ankle joint dorsiflexion increases to normal range with the knee flexed, an isolated gastrocnemius equinus is present. If ankle joint dorsiflexion is decreased with both the knee flexed and extended, a gastrocnemius-soleus equinus is present.

been ruled out by radiographic evaluation. If one considers the timing of passive ankle joint dorsiflexion in the gait cycle, this test is flawed somewhat, as the knee is relatively extended until the heel comes off the ground during toe off. Aronow and colleagues [15] performed a mechanical loading study using 10 fresh frozen cadaveric legs that were loaded with 79 lbs of plantar force through the isolated gastrocnemius, isolated soleus, or combined gastrocnemius–soleus muscles and found similar redistribution of plantar force from the rear foot to the midfoot and forefoot in each of the three muscle sets tested. These findings suggest that there is no clinically significant difference between an isolated gastrocnemius equinus and a gastrocnemius–soleus equinus, which would render the findings of the Silfverskiold test irrelevant in procedure selection. There are, however, several other reasons why one procedure would be preferable to another for an individual patient (Table 1).

Table 1
Procedure selection criteria for equinus correction

Indications for percutaneous tendo-Achilles lengthening	Indications for open gastrocnemius recession	Indications for endoscopic gastrocnemius recession
Spastic equinus	Nonspastic equinus	Nonspastic equinus
Severe deformity	Athlete requiring	No peripheral
Peripheral arterial disease	propulsive strength	arterial disease
Status post peripheral	No peripheral	Athlete requiring
bypass surgery	arterial disease	propulsive strength
Varicosities present	Varicosities absent	Inability to remain
Capable of postoperative	Inability to remain	nonweight bearing
nonweight bearing	nonweight bearing	Previous Achilles tendon
	Previous Achilles	surgery
	tendon surgery	Cosmesis

Percutaneous tendo–Achilles lengthening

Percutaneous tendo–Achilles lengthening (PTAL) is preferred in patients who have peripheral arterial disease or peripheral arterial bypass surgery because of the minimum length of the incisions required to properly complete the procedure with a low risk of primary wound healing complications [6]. Additionally, a greater degree of equinus correction can be obtained with a PTAL than an OGR or EGR, making it ideal for correcting severe equinus deformity [12,16]. Use of the PTAL procedure is necessary in conjunction with partial foot amputations at or proximal to the level of Lisfranc's joint to weaken the posterior calf musculature adequately to prevent excessive pressure on the significantly shortened foot. The patient must be able to remain nonweight bearing for 4 to 6 weeks after a PTAL procedure to limit the potential for overlengthening as a result of partial or complete rupture postoperatively [17,18]. Limited early weight bearing in a robust short-leg cast is allowed for some patients with spastic equinus contracture associated with neuromuscular disease [19,20], as these patients may benefit from slightly more length than was achieved on the operating table. Overlengthening can result in a calcaneal gait and a plantar central heel ulcer that is difficult or impossible to remedy (Fig. 2) [6,18,21–23]. There is also a risk of damage to the tibial nerve medially, the flexor hallucis longus tendon anterior–medially, and the sural nerve laterally with poor surgical technique [6,17]. Patients who have intratendinous Achilles tendon pathology are not good candidates for PTAL because of the increased risk of rupture inherent to incisions through hypovascular tendon [24,25]. The procedure additionally results in a loss of muscle mass that is cosmetically unappealing and functionally disruptive.

Open gastrocnemius recession

OGR is indicated for patients who require maintenance of the strength of the soleus muscle [8,10]. This includes athletes requiring greater propulsive strength to participate in their sport and may include patients with neurologic

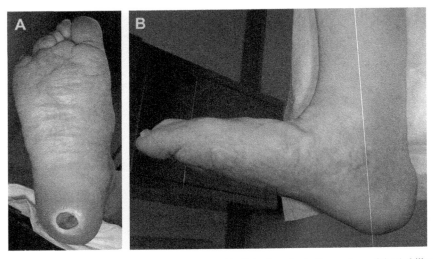

Fig. 2. Plantar central heel ulcer (*A*) in a neuropathic diabetic patient after rupture of the Achilles tendon status after percutaneous tendo-Achilles lengthening (*B*).

conditions causing postural instability, such as cerebral palsy (CP) [26,27] to avoid postoperative crouch during stance. Some authors refute this, finding similar results between PTAL and OGR in patients who have CP [20,28,29]. OGR, when performed in isolation, allows for immediate postoperative weight bearing in a protective walking boot or cast and is therefore a good choice for patients who might have difficulty remaining nonweight bearing. Additionally, there is a lower risk of overlengthening or rupture with this procedure when compared with the PTAL, unless the deep soleal fibers are released, and the aponeurosis is elevated off of the underlying musculature aggressively [6]. Tennis leg is another potential complication of the procedure resulting from dissection of the medial head of the gastrocnemius muscle off of the gastrocnemius aponeurosis, which can result in functional weakness and muscle atrophy. Injury to the lesser saphenous vein or sural nerve is a potential complication of OGR [10,30], particularly with a direct posterior approach. Patients who have varicosities also may have an increased risk of hematoma formation, because dilated, friable veins may be harder to avoid and hemostasis difficult to achieve. In patients who are morbidly obese, determining the appropriate tissue planes may be challenging, resulting in a greater likelihood of neurovascular injury and requiring a larger incision to properly visualize relevant anatomy. This increases the risk of necrosis of the adipose tissue with a resultant higher incidence of wound-healing complications.

Endoscopic gastrocnemius recession

EGR has similar indications to OGR but may be preferred in some instances, because it requires a smaller incision, resulting in a more cosmetic appearance postoperatively [10]. Additionally, the procedure may be less traumatic with a lower likelihood of hematoma formation. Use of the endoscope allows direct visualization and, therefore, protection of the sural nerve and lesser saphenous vein. The entire gastrocnemius aponeurosis also can be seen, ensuring complete transection during the procedure [10]. A thigh or sterile high calf tourniquet is required to ensure a bloodless field, which prevents the endoscope from becoming obscured. The use of a tourniquet is contraindicated in patients who have a history of peripheral arterial disease or peripheral arterial bypass surgery and is not well tolerated by the patient without the use of spinal or general anesthetic. EGR has the same potential complications as OGR.

Surgical techniques

Multiple publications regarding the surgical techniques for PTAL, OGR, and EGR exist, with varying recommendations regarding incision placement and the amount of dorsiflexion that should be achieved intraoperatively. The following techniques include the pearls provided to the author during postgraduate fellowship training (Thomas S. Roukis, DPM, FACFAS, personal communication, 2006) to aid in performance of these procedures and avoid complications associated with them.

Percutaneous tendo–Achilles lengthening

The PTAL is performed with the patient supine. The drape should be placed above the knee to facilitate application of a splint or cast postoperatively. The foot can be positioned on the surgeon's chest and dorsiflexed to apply tension to the Achilles tendon. Alternatively, an assistant can flex the knee, externally rotate the hip, and dorsiflex the foot to allow visualization of the Achilles tendon by the surgeon.

Multiple anatomic considerations have led to the use of incisions placed at 2 cm, 5 cm, and 8 cm proximal to the Achilles tendon insertion as the authors' preferred method of performing the PTAL (Fig. 3). The watershed area of the Achilles tendon is from 2 to 6 cm proximal to its insertion and is an area of relative avascularity that is highly susceptible to rupture [31,32]. Incisions are placed at the extremes of the watershed area to promote healing and 3 cm apart to reduce the risk of tendon disruption [33]. The most distal portion of the Achilles tendon is very thin and narrow and therefore susceptible to rupture or transection of more than half of the tendon fibers. The tendon becomes more substantial at 2 cm proximal to its insertion, making this a good location for incision placement. This incision is also proximal enough to maintain the heel contour, reducing the likelihood of irritation on the heel counter of the shoe [34], and allows access to the plantaris tendon medially. The plantaris tendon can be transected at this level to aide in equinus correction, if required.

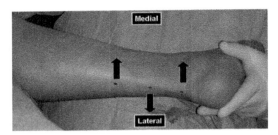

Fig. 3. Assistant positioning the leg for performance of the percutaneous tendo-Achilles length-ening with the knee flexed, the hip externally rotated, and the foot dorsiflexed to allow complete visualization of the posterior ankle and leg. Note the proper incision placement (*surgical scribe marks*) for the standard percutaneous tendo-Achilles lengthening at 2 cm, 5 cm, and 8 cm prox-imal to the Achilles tendon insertion. The black arrows demonstrate the direction of partial tendon transection.

A No. 64 beaver blade or a No.11 blade is preferred to perform the pro-cedure. An initial percutaneous stab incision is performed in a longitudinal direction at the center of the Achilles tendon 2 cm proximal to its insertion onto the calcaneus. The longitudinal incision is preferred, as it will not gap when ankle dorsiflexion is performed to lengthen the tendon. The blade should advance only through the Achilles tendon proper. The blade is turned medially to transect the medial half of the tendon, which helps to cor-rect any frontal plane hindfoot deformity (ie, varus) present [11]. A second longitudinal stab incision is made 3 cm proximal to the first with the blade turned laterally to incise the lateral half of the Achilles tendon, and then a third stab incision is made 3 cm proximal to the second for transection of the medial half of the tendon. The knee is extended, and the foot is held off the operating room table by the surgeon with the fingers intertwined over the anterior aspect of the ankle and the thumbs pushing up on the plan-tar aspect of the midfoot (Fig. 4A) while the ankle is rotated into a con-trolled dorsiflexion (see Fig. 4B), with the goal of the foot reaching 90° to the leg (see Fig. 4C). Excessive force should not be applied to dorsiflex the foot (ie, leaning into the foot with the surgeon's chest (see Fig. 4D) or forcefully pushing the foot into dorsiflexion multiple times (see Fig. 4E)). The Achilles tendon will not be healed completely when the patient begins to ambulate at 4 to 6 weeks postoperatively, allowing additional length to be obtained and thereby adding to the final correction. The desired result is between 0° and 5° of passive ankle dorsiflexion with the knee fully extended. Overlengthening may result in a calcaneal gait and development of a plantar central heel ulcer, especially in a neuropathic patient, which fre-quently will lead to lower limb amputation [35].

If the desired correction of the equinus deformity has not been achieved, each incision site should be re-evaluated to determine if adequate transec-tion of the tendon has been accomplished in the same manner as described

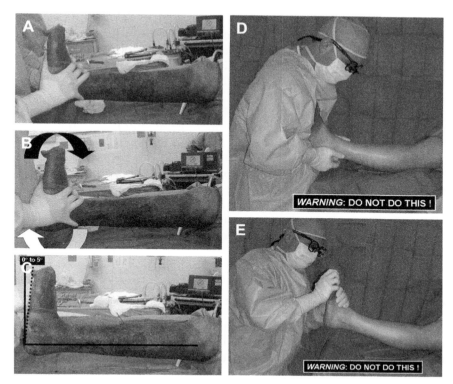

Fig. 4. After performance of the posterior lengthening procedure, controlled dorsiflexion is performed with the knee straight and foot and leg held off the bed while the fingers are intertwined at the anterior ankle (*A*). Steady pressure in a dorsal direction by the surgeon's thumbs across the midfoot is used to rotate the ankle into a corrected position (*B*). The ideal final corrected position is when passive ankle dorsiflexion is between 0° and 5° (*C*). It should be noted that each of the previously mentioned scenarios occurs with the foot at 90° to the lower leg. Excessive force, such as leaning into the foot with the surgeon's chest (*D*) or forcefully pushing on the foot multiple times (*E*) should be avoided to limit the potential for iatrogenic overlengthening or acute rupture of the tendon intraoperatively.

previously. If significant deformity continues, additional incisions can be made at 1 cm intervals between each of the original incision sites, cutting alternating portions of the lateral and medial third of the tendon. Be aware that this will increase the risk of tendon rupture postoperatively because of the added number of incisions within the tendon with a greater likelihood of violating the watershed area. The surgeon should begin with two incisions between the initial distal and middle stab incision sites. Once completed, controlled dorsiflexion should be performed again at the ankle joint. If adequate correction has been achieved, the procedure is complete. If not, two additional incisions can be made between the original middle and proximal incisions as described previously. At this point, controlled dorsiflexion again is attempted. If these maneuvers fail to provide ideal correction, consideration should be given to performing an OGR as will be described, in addition to evaluating the posterior ankle capsule for possible contracture that may prevent reduction of deformity. Skin staples can be used to close each individual incision site, with the foot held in corrected position during application.

The patient then generally is placed into a sugar tong plaster splint, which allows proper immobilization of the midfoot, hindfoot, and ankle, and should be applied with the foot held at 90° to the lower leg. The patient must remain non-weight bearing on the operated side for 4 to 6 weeks or longer depending on what additional procedures are performed. In patients who have peripheral arterial disease or status postperipheral arterial bypass surgery, where postoperative splinting is contraindicated, alternative immobilization of the ankle joint with percutaneous placement of extra-articular Steinmann pins during tendon healing can be performed, as has been described previously [36,37].

Open gastrocnemius recession

OGR is performed with the patient supine and the lower leg externally rotated. Incision placement is determined by marking out the medial aspect of the knee joint and the distal edge of the medial malleolus. The medial aspect of the lower leg is divided into thirds between these two anatomic markers. The incision is placed at the middle of the middle one third of the medial aspect of the lower leg, 2 cm posterior to the posterior most edge of the medial face of the tibia (Fig. 5A). The location can be verified by palpating the medial head of the gastrocnemius muscle (see Fig. 5B), with the incision located just distal to this structure. A 3 cm linear incision is made in this location with a No.10 blade. A hemostat then is placed into the incision and opened in line with the incision site. Care should be taken to avoid disruption of crossing veins that are often present traversing the incision site, which can obscure the operative field. Subcutaneous adipose tissue is swept aside with a moist sponge and the surgeon's index finger. Wide retractors are placed at the edges of the incision, and the deep fascia is visualized. A No.10 blade is used to incise through the deep fascia in line with the skin incision, exposing the underlying gastrocnemius aponeurosis, which then also is incised in the same manner (Fig. 6A). A tissue elevator is passed from medial-to-lateral, identifying the plane between the gastrocnemius aponeurosis and deep fascia (see Fig. 6B), until it is palpated on the lateral side of the leg. As the elevator is removed, it is swept from distal to proximal in a windshield wiper fashion to further define this plane. The wide retractors then are repositioned deep to the deep fascia to fully visualize the underlying gastrocnemius aponeurosis, and a large scissor is used to transect the gastrocnemius aponeurosis from medial-to-lateral (see Fig. 6C). The

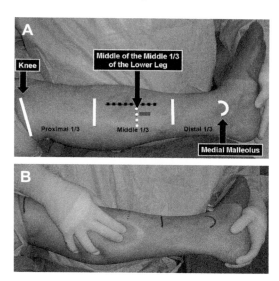

Fig. 5. Landmarks for the open gastrocnemius recession incision are shown with the medial aspect of the leg divided into thirds between the knee joint and the medial malleolus. The incision is placed at the middle of the middle one third of the leg, 2 cm posterior to the posterior edge of the medial face of the tibia (*A*). The location is verified by palpating the medial head of the gastrocnemius muscle (surgeon's index and middle finger) with the incision placed directly distal to this structure (*B*).

plantaris tendon is identified easily as the most medial structure along the medial edge of the gastrocnemius aponeurosis and is transected when visualized. A small portion of the remaining aponeurosis can be visualized at the antero–medial edge of the incision site (see Fig. 6D) and also should be transected with a large scissor, with care taken to avoid injury to the great saphenous nerve and vein that course in close proximity to the tibia at this level of the lower leg (see Fig. 6E). Controlled dorsiflexion of the foot is performed with the knee straight as described in the PTAL procedure, with a goal of getting the foot at 90° to the lower leg. The surgical site is inspected to make certain complete recession of the gastrocnemius aponeurosis has occurred (see Fig. 6F). The incision site then is irrigated with sterile saline, and the calf is compressed to exsanguinate any blood from the surgical site to prevent hematoma formation. An absorbable suture is used to close the deep fascia to avoid adhesion of the skin to the underlying tissues, which can create an unsightly dell at the incision site. The skin is closed with vertical mattress sutures of 2-0 nylon and metallic skin staples. If the procedure is performed in isolation, the patient may be placed into a weight-bearing short-leg boot or walking cast that is kept in place with the foot at 90° to the lower leg for 2 to 4 weeks.

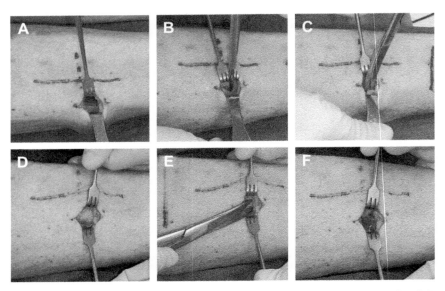

Fig. 6. Incision through the gastrocnemius aponeurosis with the deep fascia retracted and the underlying soleus muscle visualized (*A*). A tissue elevator is passed between the deep fascia and the gastrocnemius aponeurosis to create a safe tissue plane for recession (*B*). A large scissor is advanced to its hub about the gastrocnemius aponeurosis with one blade superficial to the soleus and the other deep to the deep fascia before transection (*C*). Remaining medial fibers of the gastrocnemius aponeurosis are visualized (*D*) and transected with a large scissor (*E*), with care taken to avoid injury to the great saphenous vein and nerve. Completion of the open gastrocnemius recession with visualized soleal muscle fibers (*F*).

Endoscopic gastrocnemius recession

EGR must be performed with a thigh or sterile high calf tourniquet, as bleeding during the procedure will obscure visualization through the endoscope. The patient is positioned supine with feet at the end of the table, and a stack of towels is placed posterior to the ankle to facilitate passage of instrumentation and dorsiflexion of the ankle during the procedure. The arthroscopy tower is positioned on the contralateral side of the operative limb for easy viewing during the procedure. Care must be taken to avoid knee hyperextension when assessing ankle joint dorsiflexion, as it may limit motion. A second arm board positioned at the end of the bed, on which the contralateral foot can be placed, provides additional room for the endoscopic equipment (Fig. 7A).

An incision of approximately 1 cm in length is required for the EGR and is mapped out in the same manner as for the OGR. A No. 10 blade is used to incise the skin, followed by dissection to the level of the deep fascia as described for the OGR, and incision through this structure to expose the gastrocnemius aponeurosis. The aponeurosis is incised with a No. 10 blade and a fascial elevator (A.M. Surgical Endoscopic Tissue Release, Wright Medical Technology, Incorporated, Arlington, Tennessee) is used to define the plane between the deep fascia and the gastrocnemius aponeurosis from medial-to-lateral (see Fig. 7B). A sweeping motion again is used as discussed previously during removal of the elevator. The obturator and cannula (A.M. Surgical Endoscopic Tissue Release, Wright Medical Technology, Incorporated) are inserted into this plane. The cannula is rotated so that its opening is toward the aponeurosis, and the obturator is removed (see Fig. 7C). A 4 mm, 25° to 30° endoscope is inserted (see Fig. 7D) and slowly advanced from medial-to-lateral to visualize the gastrocnemius aponeurosis and confirm that the cannula is in the correct plane.

The cannula and endoscope then are rotated posteriorly toward the deep fascia. Additionally, the endoscope is withdrawn from lateral-to-medial to visualize the lesser saphenous vein and sural nerve, which frequently do not course in close proximity to each other, to ensure that the cannula lies anterior to these structures to prevent injury to them (see Fig. 7E). Once confirmed, the endoscope and cannula are rotated back 180°, so the opening again faces the gastrocnemius aponeurosis. The endoscope is removed, and the endoscope-mounted knife blade (A.M. Surgical Endoscopic Tissue Release, Wright Medical Technology, Incorporated) is applied to the endoscope and locked in place (see Fig. 7F). The endoscope and knife blade are inserted into the cannula, being careful not to inadvertently incise the skin during entry. The foot is dorsiflexed and the cannula angled slightly toward the gastrocnemius aponeurosis (see Fig. 7G) while the endoscope and knife blade are advanced with both hands in a controlled fashion from medial-to-lateral, incising the aponeurosis (see Fig. 7H). On initiation of the incision, the endoscope and knife blade can be twisted gently from side-to-side to properly engage and begin transecting the medial fibers of the gastrocnemius aponeurosis. Then the instrumentation generally can be advanced through the aponeurosis without significant resistance to complete the release. A stopper on the blade prevents extrusion through the skin at the lateral aspect of the lower leg.

To increase contact between the knife blade and gastrocnemius aponeurosis, the surgeon or his or her assistant can push anteriorly on the posterior calf overlying the cannula while the blade is advanced (see Fig. 7I). The endoscope and knife blade then are removed slowly while the surgeon confirms that complete transection has been accomplished. This is evidenced by visualization of the soleus muscle fibers through the transected edges of the gastrocnemius aponeurosis along its entire course from medial-to-lateral. If portions of the gastrocnemius aponeurosis remain intact, the endoscope and knife blade again are passed through the cannula to incise the remaining regions, being careful not to incise the underlying muscle fibers, which can create excessive bleeding and cause hematoma formation. If visualization becomes obscured at any point in the procedure, the endoscope can be removed and sterile cotton swabs placed through the cannula

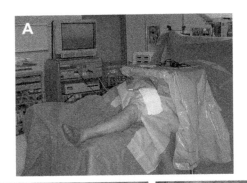

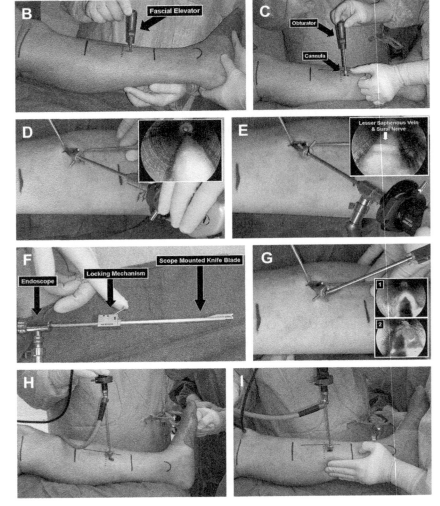

to clear the operative field. Controlled dorsiflexion of the ankle is performed to assess for correction of deformity. If the correction is inadequate, the endoscope and knife blade are removed, and irrigation is performed through the cannula. The obturator then is placed into the cannula, and both the obturator and cannula are removed to prevent trauma to the soft tissues. A large scissor is used to transect the medial most fibers of the gastrocnemius aponeurosis at the anterior border of the incision site as described previously. If additional correction is required, elevation of the gastrocnemius aponeurosis off of the underlying soleus can be achieved with a tissue elevator. Although described in the literature, use of an accessory lateral incision should be avoided to prevent iatrogenic injury to the superficial peroneal nerve, which courses through the lateral compartment of the lower leg [38]. The deep fascia is closed with absorbable suture for the reasons described previously, followed by skin closure, also described previously. If performed as an isolated procedure, the postoperative course is identical to that for the OGR.

Summary

Soft-tissue ankle equinus contracture contributes to the etiology of multiple foot disorders and must be addressed to achieve global correction of deformity. A sound understanding of the indications for each procedure, the relevant topographic anatomic landmarks for incision placement, and the operative technique will aide the surgeon in achieving the best possible results. There is potential for complications with any of the described techniques. Appropriate procedure selection for the individual patient, however, with care to avoid overlengthening in the operating room, along with protection of the involved extremity postoperatively leads to reproducible success with these procedures even in the high-risk patient.

Fig. 7. Intra-operative photograph demonstrating proper set-up for performing an endoscopic gastrocnemius recession (A). Insertion of the fascial elevator between the deep fascia and gastrocnemius aponeurosis (B). Insertion of the cannula and obturator into the developed plane superficial to the gastrocnemius aponeurosis and deep to the deep fascia (C). The cannula will remain after removing the obturator. With the cannula rotated toward the aponeurosis, a 4 mm, 25° to 30° endoscope is inserted to visualize the gastrocnemius aponeurosis across its full width from medial-to-lateral (D). Once the gastrocnemius aponeurosis has been visualized, the endoscope and cannula are rotated posteriorly toward the deep fascia to withdraw from lateral-to-medial, with care taken to identify the sural nerve and lesser saphenous vein within the adipose tissue (E). The locking mechanism is applied to the scope-mounted knife blade, and both are inserted onto the endoscope (F). The foot is held in dorsiflexion to place tension on the gastrocnemius aponeurosis by the assistant (G), and the endoscope and knife are angled toward the aponeurosis during advancement to transect the gastrocnemius aponeurosis (H). An assistant also can increase contact between the knife blade and gastrocnemius aponeurosis by pushing the cannula anteriorly on the posterior calf while the blade is advanced (I).

References

[1] Pinney SJ, Hansen ST, Sangeorzan BJ. The effect on ankle dorsiflexion of gastrocnemius recession. Foot Ankle Int 2002;23(1):26–9.

[2] Willrich A, Angirasa AK, Sage RA. Percutaneous tendo–Achilles lengthening to promote healing of diabetic plantar foot ulceration. J Am Podiatr Med Assoc 2005;95(3):281–4.

[3] Mueller MJ, Sinacore DR, Hastings MK, et al. Effect of Achilles tendon lengthening on neuropathic plantar ulcers: a randomized clinical trial. J Bone Joint Surg Am 2003;85(8): 1436–45.

[4] Armstrong DG, Stacpoole-Shea S, Nguyen H, et al. Lengthening of the Achilles tendon in diabetics who are at high risk for ulceration of the foot. J Bone Joint Surg Am 1999;81(4): 535–8.

[5] Armstrong DG, Stacpoole-Shea S, Nguyen H, et al. Lengthening of the Achilles tendon in diabetic patients. J Bone Joint Surg Am 2000;82(10):1510.

[6] Nishimoto GS, Attinger CE, Cooper PS. Lengthening the Achilles tendon for the treatment of diabetic plantar forefoot ulceration. Surg Clin North Am 2003;83(3):707–26.

[7] Tashjian RZ, Appel AJ, Banerjee R, et al. Anatomic study of the gastrocnemius–soleus junction and its relationship to the sural nerve. Foot Ankle Int 2003;24(6):473–6.

[8] Panchbhavi VK, Trevino SG. Endoscopic gastrocnemius recession. Techniques in Foot and Ankle Surgery 2004;3(3):149–52.

[9] Rush SM, Ford LA, Hamilton GA. Morbidity associated with high gastrocnemius recession: retrospective review of 126 cases. J Foot Ankle Surg 2006;45(3):156–60.

[10] Saxena A, Widtfeldt A. Endoscopic gastrocnemius recession: preliminary report on 18 cases. J Foot Ankle Surg 2004;43(5):302–6.

[11] DiDomenico LA, Adams HB, Garchar D. Endoscopic gastrocnemius recession for the treatment of gastrocnemius equinus. J Am Podiatr Med Assoc 2005;95(4):410–3.

[12] Lamm BM, Paley D, Herzenberg JE. Gastrocnemius–soleus recession: a simpler, more limited approach. J Am Podiatr Med Assoc 2005;95(1):18–25.

[13] Crawford M. Pertinent pointers on equinus procedures. Podiatr Today 2007;20(6):38–50.

[14] Kim PJ, Steinberg JS. Tendo–Achilles lengthening: friend or foe in the diabetic foot. Podiatr Today 2007;20(11):20–6.

[15] Aronow MS, Diaz-Doran V, Sullivan RJ, et al. The effect of triceps surae contracture force on plantar foot pressure distribution. Foot Ankle Int 2006;27(1):43–52.

[16] Herzenberg JE, Lamm BM, Corwin C, et al. Isolated recession of the gastrocnemius muscle: the Baumann procedure. Foot Ankle Int 2007;28(11):1154–9.

[17] Salamon ML, Pinney SJ, Bergeyk AV, et al. Surgical anatomy and accuracy of percutaneous Achilles tendon lengthening. Foot Ankle Int 2006;27(6):411–3.

[18] Haro AA, DiDomenico LA. Frontal plane-guided percutaneous tendo Achilles lengthening. J Foot Ankle Surg 2007;46(1):55–61.

[19] Meszaros A, Caudell G. The surgical management of equinus in the adult acquired flatfoot. Clin Podiatr Med Surg 2007;24(4):667–85.

[20] Greene WB. Cerebral palsy. Evaluation and management of equinus and equinovarus deformities. Foot Ankle Clin 2000;5(2):265–80.

[21] Gabarino JL, Clancy M. A geometric method of calculating tendo–Achilles lengthening. J Pediatr Orthop 1985;5(5):573–6.

[22] Costa ML, Logan K, Heylings D, et al. The effect of Achilles tendon lengthening on ankle dorsiflexion: a cadaver study. Foot Ankle Int 2006;27(6):414–7.

[23] Holstein P, Lohmann M, Bitsch M, et al. Achilles tendon lengthening, the panacea for plantar forefoot ulceration? Diabetes Metab Res Rev 2004;20(Suppl 1):S37–40.

[24] Tallon C, Maffulli N, Ewen SW. Ruptured Achilles tendons are significantly more degenerated than tendinopathic tendons. Med Sci Sports Exerc 2001;33(12):1983–90.

[25] Maffulli N, Barrass V, Ewen SW. Light microscopic histology of Achilles tendon ruptures. A comparison with unruptured tendons. Am J Sports Med 2000;28(6):857–63.

[26] Tashjian RZ, Appel AJ, Banerjee R, et al. Endoscopic gastrocnemius recession: evaluation in a cadaver model. Foot Ankle Int 2003;24(8):607–13.
[27] Sharrard WJ, Bernstein S. Equinus deformity in cerebral palsy a comparison between elongation of the tendo–calcaneus and gastrocnemius recession. J Bone Joint Surg Br 1972;54(2): 272–6.
[28] Orendurff MS, Aiona MD, Dorociak RD, et al. Length and force of the gastrocnemius and soleus during gait following tendo Achilles lengthenings in children with equinus. Gait Posture 2002;15(2):130–5.
[29] Fulford GE. Surgical management of ankle and foot deformities in cerebral palsy. Clin Orthop Relat Res 1990;253:55–61.
[30] Pinney SJ, Sangeorzan BJ, Hansen ST. Surgical anatomy of the gastrocnemius recession (Strayer procedure). Foot Ankle Int 2004;25(4):247–50.
[31] Saxena A, Bareither D. Magnetic resonance and cadaveric findings of the watershed band of the Achilles tendon. J Foot Ankle Surg 2001;40(3):132–6.
[32] Werd MB. Achilles tendon sports injuries. A review of classification and treatment. J Am Podiatr Med Assoc 2007;97(1):37–48.
[33] Hoffman B, Nunley J. Achilles tendon torsion has no effect on percutaneous triple-cut tenotomy results. Foot Ankle Int 2006;27(11):960–4.
[34] Sammarco GJ, Bagwe MR, Sammarco J, et al. The effects of unilateral gastrocsoleus recession. Foot Ankle Int 2006;27(7):508–11.
[35] Chilvers M, Malicky ES, Anderson JG, et al. Heel overload associated with heel cord insufficiency. Foot Ankle Int 2007;28(6):687–9.
[36] League A, Parks B, Öznur A, et al. Transarticular versus extra-articular ankle pin fixation: a biomechanical study. Foot Ankle Int 2008;29(1):62–5.
[37] Schweinberger MH, Roukis TS. Extra-articular immobilization for protection of percutaneous tendo–Achilles lengthening following transmetatarsal amputation and peripheral arterial bypass surgery. J Foot Ankle Surg 2008;47(2):169–71.
[38] Ducic I, Dellon AL, Graw KS. The clinical importance of variations in the surgical anatomy of the superficial peroneal nerve in the midthird of the lateral leg. Ann Plast Surg 2006;56(6): 635–8.

ELSEVIER
SAUNDERS

Clin Podiatr Med Surg
25 (2008) 587–607

CLINICS IN
PODIATRIC
MEDICINE AND
SURGERY

Minimum-Incision Metatarsal Osteotomies

Thomas S. Roukis, DPM, FACFAS*,
Valerie L. Schade, DPM, AACFAS

*Limb Preservation Service, Vascular/Endovascular Surgery Service,
Department of Surgery, Madigan Army Medical Center,
9040-A Fitzsimmons Avenue, MCHJ-SV, Tacoma, WA 98431, USA*

Minimum-incision surgery is defined as surgery performed through the smallest incision necessary to perform the procedure properly, while percutaneous surgery is defined as surgery performed within the smallest possible working incision without direct visualization of the deeper structures [1]. When performed properly by experienced surgeons for appropriate conditions, both of these techniques allow for limited surgical trauma to the surrounding tissues and maximum alternation of anatomic structures [1]. The field of plastic and reconstructive surgery was the modern origin of these techniques, using minimal incision approaches to remove and remodel bones in a limited exposure fashion to minimize visible scars.

In 1945, Morton Polokoff was the first podiatric physician to employ subdermal surgery using very fine chisels, rasps, and spears. The motivation for these approaches at the time was to enhance the surgical capabilities of podiatric physicians by circumventing restrictive laws regarding surgery for podiatric physicians at that time [2]. Minimum-incision approaches originally were performed in the office setting to treat minor forefoot abnormalities as an ambulatory procedure [2]. Edwin Probber introduced larger instrumentation for these procedures in the 1960s with Bernard Weinstock using the earliest power equipment [2,3]. Minimum-incision rear foot procedures consisting of plantar calcaneal spur resections also started at this time [2]. In 1972,

The opinions or assertions contained herein are the private views of the author and are not to be construed as official or reflecting the views of the Department of the Army or the Department of Defense.

* Corresponding author.

E-mail address: thomas.s.roukis@us.army.mil (T.S. Roukis).

0891-8422/08/$ - see front matter. Published by Elsevier Inc.
doi:10.1016/j.cpm.2008.05.007

Michael Perrone was the first to publish a book regarding these minimum-incision and percutaneous foot surgeries, in which he described the use of power rotary burrs [2]. Leonard Britton was the first to perform percutaneous first metatarsal opening, closing, and dorsiflexory wedge and Akin osteotomies to treat bunion deformities [2]. In 1974, minimum-incision and percutaneous procedures become part of the curriculum at the Pennsylvania College of Podiatric Medicine [2,3] and were advanced further with the introduction of the low-intensity radiographic imaging scope (ie, Lixiscope) [4]. O.T. New discussed the technique he employed to perform a subcutaneous resection of a first metatarsal pseudoexostosis with Peter Bösch in 1983 [5]. The following year, Bösch began performing a percutaneous or subcutaneous metatarsal first osteotomy (SCOT) with a power burr, which he termed the "subcutaneous Bösch technique" as his treatment of choice for surgical correction of the hallux valgus deformity [5]. The osteotomy employed a Hohmann-type configuration [6] and was fixated with an axial Steinmann pin as described by Lamprecht and Kramer [7] in 1982. It is worth noting that podiatric physicians were employing nearly identical procedures before these publications; however, the osteotomies were not fixated. Instead an elaborate dressing was employed to maintain alignment and provide stability until the osteotomies became sound by means of secondary osseous healing, usually with exuberant osseous callus formation [8,9]. Giannini performed essentially the same procedure as that described by Bösch. He, however, employed a 1 cm incision and used a power saw blade rather than a rotary burr, thereby employing a minimum incision technique that he summarized as simple, effective, rapid, and inexpensive (SERI) [10]. Numerous manuscripts have been published describing essentially the same percutaneous and minimum-incision approaches described previously for correction of the hallux valgus deformity with near universal success [5,11–17]. Most complications reported appear to be a direct result of poor surgical technique [18–20]. In reviewing the manuscripts published by authors who encountered significant complications attempting to employ percutaneous or minimum-incision approaches to surgical correction of the hallux valgus deformity, it becomes clear that the surgeons either:

Unwisely modified established techniques
Performed the procedures using a traditional open incision
Had limited formal training or experience performing percutaneous and minimum- incision surgery about the forefoot [18–20].

In contrast to the literature discussing the use of percutaneous and minimum-incision techniques for surgical correction of the hallux valgus deformity, use of these techniques for pathology about the central metatarsals has received comparatively little attention in the literature [21–23]. Similarly, use of these techniques for pathology about the fifth metatarsal also has received little attention [21,22,24–27].

Percutaneous and minimum-incision metatarsal osteotomies mandate a sound understanding of traditional open procedures and have a steep learning curve associated with them, because these procedures are performed in a blind or closed fashion (ie, percutaneous) or with limited visualization capability (ie, minimum incision) [1]. Intraoperative image intensification enhances the surgeon's capability to perform these techniques but is not a substitute for surgeon experience. It is interesting to note the use of components of the SCOT and SERI with traditional open procedures such as the use of the axial intramedullary buttress Steinmann pin to stabilize the metatarsal head following osteotomy [28] and the recent popularity of nonosteotomy techniques to reduce the intermetatarsal 1-2 angle associated with the hallux valgus deformity [29,30].

It seems intuitive that percutaneous and minimum-incision techniques would be beneficial in the high-risk patient with an ulceration or recurrent ulceration as a means of performing limb preservation/salvage without extensive soft-tissue and osseous trauma. This, however, has been mentioned only briefly in the literature [23–25]. Traditionally, emphasis has been placed on the use of conservative measures to relieve pressure and shear about forefoot ulcerations [31–37]. The literature does support this approach to heal forefoot ulcerations, however, because the most likely cause for developing the ulcer was a structural foot deformity, usually combined with some degree of peripheral sensory neuropathy [38–41]. It is difficult, therefore, to keep these ulcerations healed with conservative efforts [42]. There is emerging evidence that in select cases, realignment of the mechanical forefoot deformities associated with the high-risk patient decreases the need for chronic wound care and improves outcome [43]. The senior author (TSR) routinely employs percutaneous soft-tissue and minimum-incision osseous techniques to perform forefoot realignment in the high-risk patient who is determined to be unlikely to heal with traditional surgical approaches and otherwise would undergo a toe or partial foot amputation or suffer from repeated ulceration as a result of significant structural pathology incapable of being managed with conservative measures. This is the focus of the current article and not patients who would be served best with traditional open surgical approaches, because indiscriminate use of percutaneous and minimum-incision procedures in the general public can lead to significant complications (Fig. 1). Therefore, this article discusses:

The specific minimum-incision techniques used to treat hallux valgus deformities with associated toe ulceration(s) (Fig. 2)

Central and fifth metatarsal osteotomies to surgically off-load plantar ulcerative lesions recalcitrant to conservative wound healing modalities or recurrent despite these treatments (Fig. 3)

The soft-tissue and osseous vascular supply for the forefoot

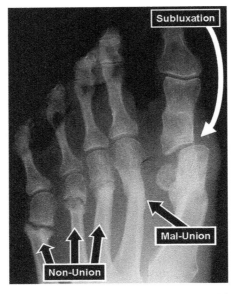

Fig. 1. Anterior–posterior weight-bearing radiograph following multiple metatarsal osteotomies performed by an inexperienced surgeon using percutaneous techniques in a patient not considered at high risk. Note the associated resultant deformities at each osteotomy. The authors advocate that percutaneous and minimum-incision techniques should be reserved for high-risk patients who are unable to undergo traditional open surgical procedures.

First metatarsal vascular supply

The extraosseous vascular supply to the first metatarsal and the first metatarsophalangeal joint occurs by means of three main vessels:

1. The first dorsal metatarsal artery, arising from the dorsalis pedis artery as it courses plantar at the base of the first metatarsal
2. The first plantar metatarsal artery arising from the deep perforating branch of the dorsalis pedis artery in the proximal first intermetatarsal space
3. An inconsistent branch of the medial plantar artery [44]

The first dorsal metatarsal artery travels distally in the first intermetatarsal space superficially, through or deep to the dorsal interosseous muscle and supplies branches primarily to the dorsal and lateral aspect of the first metatarsophalangeal joint. The plantar metatarsal artery supplies the plantar and lateral aspect of the first metatarsophalangeal joint. The inconsistent branch of the medial plantar artery supplies the plantar and medial aspects of the joint. These three primary vessels form a plantar cruciate anastomosis or extracapsular ring at the neck of the first metatarsal. Shereff and colleagues [44] determined the first dorsal metatarsal artery to be the principle

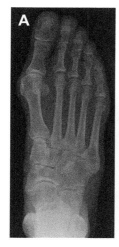
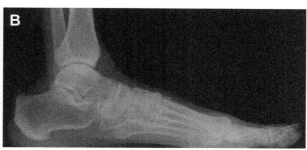

Fig. 2. Anterior–posterior (*A*) and lateral (*B*) weight-bearing radiographs and anterior–posterior (*C*) and en fass (*D*) clinical images of a patient considered high risk as a result of peripheral vascular insufficiency with a drop foot deformity who presented with a full-thickness ulceration and septic second toe proximal interphalangeal joint (*E*) as a result of direct pressure from the hallux associated with his large hallux valgus deformity. Initial treatment consisted of in-patient management employing a multidisciplinary approach and resection of the infected soft tissue and bone about the second toe with insertion of polymethylmethacrylate antibiotic-loaded bone cement into the defect. In a staged fashion, reconstruction of the second toe was performed using autogenous bone graft harvested from the lateral calcaneus (*F*), which was covered with a random-pattern Rhomboid flap (*G*). A derotational, varisation Akin-type osteotomy then was performed through a 1.5 cm Z-shaped incision and fixated with a single compression staple to correct the valgus alignment to the hallux and remove pressure against the second toe, which was the cause of the ulceration (*H*). Intraoperative simulated weight-bearing radiographs following the previously mentioned surgeries revealed incomplete reduction of the deformity (*I*), and a minimum-incision first metatarsal osteotomy was deemed necessary. Intraoperative image intensification demonstrating the location and orientation of a Steinmann pin inserted as described in the text before (*J*) and after osteotomy (*K*), as well as during the pull-and-push maneuver discussed in the text (*L*). Anterior–posterior (*M*) and lateral (*N*) intraoperative image intensification views following completion of the procedures discussed demonstrating appropriate reduction of the deformities and stable fixation. Note that the first metatarsal osteotomy was performed slightly proximal to the ideal location discussed in the text but that slight dorsal displacement was a desired effect because of the patient's drop foot deformity and preulcerative lesion at the plantar medial first metatarsal head. Anterior–posterior (*O*) and medial (*P*) clinical views 5 days postoperatively identifying the location and nature of the surgical procedures performed. Weight-bearing anterior–posterior (*Q*), en fass (*R*), and medial (*S*) clinical photographs following complete healing of each surgical procedure revealing appropriate realignment and preservation of the second toe. Weight-bearing anterior–posterior (*T*) and lateral (*U*) radiographs following complete healing of the surgical procedures demonstrating primary incorporation of the autogenous calcaneal bone graft into the resected second toe site and primary osseous healing of both the hallux and first metatarsal osteotomies with maintained alignment. Note that the first metatarsal osteotomy has remained in the same position when compared with the intraoperative images, indicating sound fixation and the location of the calcaneal bone graft harvest. which was back-filled with synthetic bone graft material (Prodense, Wright Medical Technology, Incorporated, Arlington, Tennessee) to provide immediate structural support.

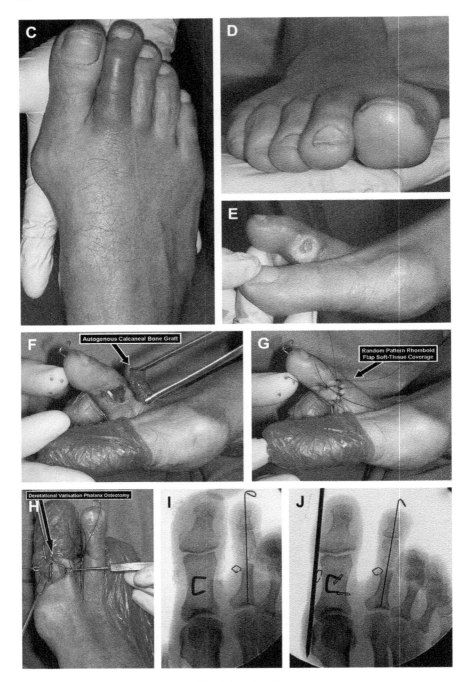

Fig. 2 (continued)

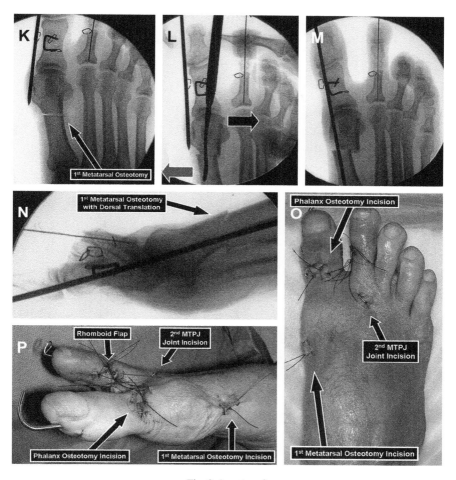

Fig. 2 (*continued*)

artery supplying the first metatarsophalangeal joint. The intraosseous vascular supply to the first metatarsal and the first metatarsophalangeal joint consists of:

Periosteal arterial supply, which enters at the diaphyseal cortex

A single nutrient artery, entering at the lateral cortical junction of the middle and distal third of the metatarsal shaft

The metaphyseal–capital arteries entering at the dorsal–medial and dorsal–lateral aspect [44]

Minimum-incision first metatarsal osteotomy: surgical technique

The surgical technique begins with the patient positioned in a supine position on the operating room table. A tourniquet is not required, as the

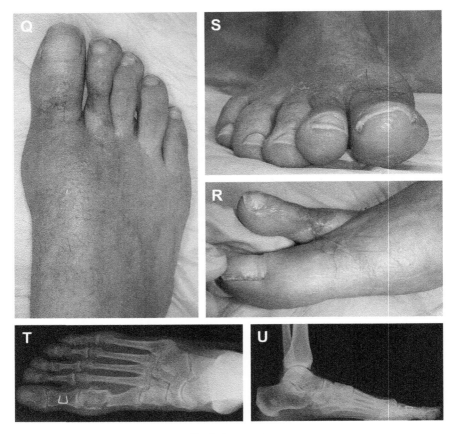

Fig. 2 (*continued*)

expected blood loss is minimal because of the limited soft-tissue dissection required for this procedure, which is reserved for the high-risk patient where use of a tourniquet also would be contraindicated. Following regional infiltration of local anesthesia and monitored intravenous sedation, intraoperative image intensification is employed to create a 1 cm vertical incision just proximal to the medial eminence of the first metatarsal at the level of the metaphyseal–diaphyseal junction (ie, subcapital region), equidistant between the dorsal and plantar aspects of the underlying first metatarsal. The periosteum is incised parallel to the longitudinal axis of the first metatarsal, and a small periosteal elevator or hemostat is inserted to reflect the periosteum off of the dorsal, medial, and plantar aspects of the first metatarsal. Following reflection of the periosteum, small angled retractors are placed within the incision to allow visualization of the first metatarsal. A 2 mm Steinmann-pin is inserted into the distal medial aspect of the hallux plantar to the nail plate and advanced proximally directly overlying the periosteum of the distal and proximal phalanges of the hallux. At the level of the first metatarsophalangeal joint, the hallux is held in a slightly overcorrected position (ie, varus), and the pin is advanced adjacent to the medial eminence of the first metatarsal head until the tip is visualized at the distal edge of the incision described previously (Fig. 2J). A narrow-width (ie, 5mm), long sagittal saw blade then is placed slightly proximal to the metaphyseal–diaphyseal junction of the first metatarsal under intraoperative image intensification control. The osteotomy should be oriented 90° to the long axis of the second metatarsal and plantar weight-bearing surface of the foot, which will allow strict lateral translation. The osteotomy is made from medial-to-lateral, with care taken not to violate the lateral cortex to prevent iatrogenic injury to the vascular supply about the first intermetatarsal space. This is different from the technique described by Giannini and colleagues [10], which most closely matches the overall technique the authors employ. A small osteotome then is inserted into the osteotomy site and rotated in controlled fashion to complete the osteotomy (Fig. 2K). It should be noted that the use of the saw allows for precise and rapid creation of the osteotomy, which the senior author (TSR) has been unable to reproduce with use of a power burr in the time frame necessary to limit complications associated with thermal injury [45]. Using the Steinmann pin and hallux as a toggle, the capital fragment is mobilized with a laterally directed force until displacement is deemed appropriate based on clinical reduction and intraoperative image intensification evaluation. It is frequently necessary to apply a medially directed force on the remaining first metatarsal with the use of a periosteal elevator within the medullary canal, which functions as a lever at the same time as lateral displacement of the capital fragment similar to the pull-and-push technique described by Barouk [46] (Fig. 2L). Care must be taken not to displace the capital fragment within the intermetatarsal space and to avoid unwanted sagittal and frontal plane deviations of the capital fragment. Once displacement is deemed appropriate, the Steinmann pin is inserted within medullary canal of the first metatarsal (Fig. 2M) and into the dense subchondral bone of the first metatarsal (Fig. 2N). The hallux should be in slight varus upon completion of fixation (Fig. 2O). The surgical site then is irrigated, and the skin is closed with a single vertical mattress suture of 2-0 nylon and metallic skin staples. The distal tip of the Steinman pin is bent carefully and cut, remaining external at that distal tip of the hallux, where it is wrapped with petroleum-impregnated gauze to limit pin site irritation and infection (Fig. 2P). A bulky, well-padded dressing from toes-to-knee then is applied [47]. The patient is placed into a post-operative shoe (Med-Surg, Darco International, Incorporated, Huntington, West Virginia) with a low-profile rocker sole and orthosis system (Peg-Assist, Darco International, Incorporated) that consists of layers of varying density and heat-moldable liners with a series of removable pegs that enhance shock absorption and off-loading, respectively. The initial surgical dressings are

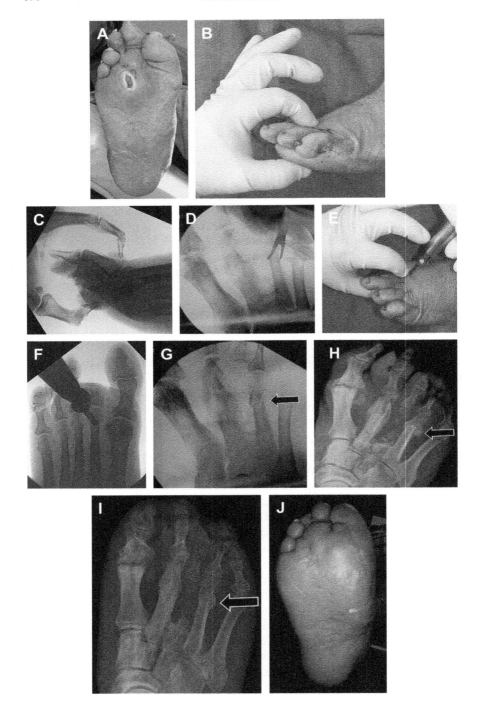

removed in 5 to 7 days unless a wound is present that requires closer monitoring, and then every 7 to 10 days thereafter. The patient is allowed partial weight bearing with a gait aide but strictly prohibited from rolling-off of the forefoot for 6 to 8 weeks or until there is evidence of osseous callus formation about the osteotomy site (Fig. 2Q–U). Once this occurs, the Steinman pin is removed in the office under aseptic technique, and guarded full-weight bearing is initiated using the same postoperative shoe and orthosis system with a gradual return to extradepth shoe gear with accommodative multidensity insoles for life [47].

Weinberger and colleagues [9] performed a retrospective review of 301 percutaneous, unfixated first metatarsal osteotomies for treating hallux valgus that revealed a mean first metatarsal shortening of 5.8 mm ± 2.6 mm, 47 dorsal malunions (15.6%), 11 infections (3.7%), seven second metatarsal stress fractures (2.3%), four delayed unions (1.2%), and one hallux varus (0.3%). Bösch and colleagues [5] performed his technique in 114 patients with no complications of hallux varus, pseudoarthrosis, or avascular necrosis of the first metatarsal head [9]. Portaluri [12] performed retrospective clinical and radiographic evaluation of 182 Bösch procedures with a mean follow-up of 16.4 ± 2.4 months, which revealed eight superficial infections (4.4%), two ulcerations about the hallux Steinmann pin site (1.1%), and two dorsal malunions (1.1%). Giannini and colleagues [10] performed a retrospective review of 54 minimum incision first metatarsal osteotomies and reported five (9.2%) delayed unions, four (7.5%) incidences of transfer metatarsalgia, three (5.5%) superficial inflammatory reactions around the hallux Steinman pin site, one (1.6%) deep vein thrombosis, and no nonunions or avascular necrosis. Sanna and Ruiu [14] performed a retrospective review of 52 feet treated with percutaneous distal-first metatarsal osteotomies (PDO), which was a hybrid between the techniques described by Bösch and colleagues [5] and Giannini and colleagues [10]. Over a mean follow-up

---

Fig. 3. Clinical image of a patient considered high-risk as a result of diabetes, morbid obesity, dense peripheral neuropathy, peripheral vascular insufficiency, underlying Charcot midfoot deformity, and multiple previously failed forefoot surgeries and clinical wound care trials with a full-thickness ulceration underlying the fourth metatarsal head (A). Intraoperative clinical (B) and image intensification (C) views of a different patient than noted previously, demonstrating the thumb-to-index finger maneuver as discussed in the text. Intraoperative image intensification view demonstrating use of a hemostat as discussed in the text to properly locate the underlying metatarsal to perform a minimum-incision osteotomy (D). Intraoperative clinical (E) and image intensification (F) views demonstrating proper placement of the saw blade to perform the minimum-incision central metatarsal osteotomy. Anterior–posterior immediate postoperative image intensification view (G), as well as, weight- bearing 4-week postoperative (H) and 1-year postoperative (I) radiographs demonstrating initial displacement of the capital fragment followed by proliferative osseous callus formation and final remodeling. Clinical image of the same patient shown in (A) demonstrating a well-healed and stable plantar forefoot following minimum-incision central metatarsal osteotomy (J).

period of 31.5 months, the authors reported four (7.4%) superficial infections and three (5.8%) ulcerations about the hallux Steinmann pin site, one (2%) recurrent deformity, one (2%) incidence of permanent anesthesia about the hallux, and one (2%) overlengthening of the first metatarsal [14]. Piqué-Vidal [45] performed a prospective evaluation of 94 percutaneous, unfixated first metatarsal and Akin osteotomies similar to the Bösch procedure and reported four delayed unions (4.3%) and no incidences of infection, nonunion, or avascular necrosis. Magnan and colleagues [15] performed a retrospective review of 118 Bösch procedures with: one foot having an ulcerated bunion and reported:

Eight (6.8%) incidences of first metatarsophalangeal joint arthrofibrosis
Three (2.5%) recurrent deformities
Three (2.5%) permanent anesthesia of the hallux
Two (1.7%) superficial infections
One (0.8%) deep infection

All resolved with antibiotic therapy, and no delayed unions or nonunions were reported. Viladot and colleagues [48] performed a retrospective review of 101 modified Kramer osteotomies, which are open versions of the SERI described by Giannini and colleagues [10], in 78 patients with a mean follow-up of 23.3 ± 6.9 months. The authors reported two (2.4%) superficial infections that resolved with oral antibiosis, two (2.4%) delayed unions, one (1.2%) deep infection requiring debridement, one (1.2%) deep venous thrombosis, one (1.2%) instance of extrusion of the percutaneous Kirschner wire fixation, and no instance of nonunion. Kadakia and colleagues [20] performed a prospective study comparing the traditional open Chevron osteotomy with a modified minimum-incision first metatarsal osteotomy using an altered fixation technique compared with the techniques described previously [5,10,12–17] with a mean follow-up of 130 days. The authors stopped the study after 3 months of enrollment because of the high complication rate they experienced, which included:

Nine (69%) dorsal malunions
Five (38%) recurrent deformities
One (7.7%) incidence of avascular necrosis
One (7.7%) nonunion
One (7.7%) superficial infection that resolved with antibiotic therapy.

The authors stated that because they performed the osteotomy more proximally in the metatarsal than recommended, this may have compromised the vascular supply to the osteotomy. One procedure also had an associated lateral distal soft-tissue release, which can disrupt vascular supply to the first metatarsal head [49–51] and lead to delayed union, nonunion, and avascular necrosis [52–54], although it was not mentioned if this patient was one of the patients who developed a complication. The authors had their patients' weight bearing as tolerated in a stiff-soled postoperative shoe immediately postoperatively, in contrast with the other studies where patients were weight bearing in a forefoot off-loading shoe with a kidney-shaped pad placed on the plantar foot to offload the distal first metatarsal and an elaborate stabilizing dressing [5,10,12–17]. These factors, combined with the surgeons inexperience using the specific technique intended to be studied, may explain the high number of complications in their study [20]. After reviewing the complications reported with unfixated first metatarsal osteotomies, the benefit of intramedullary axial Steinmann pin fixation in stabilizing the first metatarsal against dorsal angulation or translation following percutaneous and minimum-incision osteotomy and the specific angle of the osteotomy to limit shortening of the first metatarsal with the associated known complications is noteworthy [5,8–20]. Sagittal plane elevation of the first metatarsal and excessive shortening have a known detrimental effect on function of the first metatarsophalangeal joint and forefoot. Therefore, unless necessary to treat the structural pathology, it should be avoided by properly performing the metatarsal osteotomy and stabilizing it throughout the postoperative period [55–64].

Central metatarsal vascular supply

The vascular supply of the central metatarsals comes from the dorsal metatarsal arteries, arising from the arcuate artery, and the plantar metatarsal arteries, arising from the plantar arch of the lateral plantar artery [65,66]. The dorsal metatarsal arteries travel distal through the intermetatarsal space dorsal to the dorsal interosseous muscle to supply the dorsal aspect of the metatarsophalangeal joint. The dorsal and plantar capsular vessels anastomose to supply the metatarsal head at the level of the extra-articular dorsal synovial fold and the collateral ligament attachments. The plantar metatarsal arteries travel distal through the intermetatarsal space between the plantar interosseous and the oblique head of the adductor hallucis muscle. The plantar metatarsal arteries produce two terminal branches at the plantar metaphyseal–diaphyseal junction, proximal to the attachment of the plantar plate. One artery supplies the plantar capsular structures, including the plantar plate, and the other artery supplies the metatarsal head. The extraosseous vascular network supplying the metatarsal heads shares a rich anastomosis between the second and third metatarsals, the third and fourth metatarsals, and the fourth and fifth metatarsals. There is no anastomosis between the first and second metatarsal heads. The nutrient arteries for the metatarsal heads enter the metaphyseal cortex at the level of the capsular insertion [65,66].

Minimum-incision central metatarsal osteotomy: surgical technique

The surgical technique begins as described previously for minimum-incision osteotomy of the first metatarsal. A predictable maneuver the senior author (TSR) was taught to use [23] to identify the proper location to perform a minimum-incision central metatarsal osteotomy is to first place the thumb of the nondominant hand directly over the metatarsal head or plantar ulceration. Next, the index finger of the nondominant hand is placed over the dorsal aspect of the metatarsal in line with the thumb (Fig. 3 B). This creates an "okay" sign and identifies the proximal extent of the metatarsal surgical neck at the level of the metaphyseal–diaphyseal junction where the osteotomy should be performed (Fig. 3 C). A 1 cm transverse incision is placed through the skin at the dorsal aspect of the selected metatarsal surgical neck just proximal to the surgeon's index finger. A hemostat with the jaws fully closed then is used to dissect down to the level of the periosteum overlying the intended osteotomy. Once the bone is palpated, the hemostat jaws are opened with one jaw placed medial and the other lateral until the hemostat can be advanced from dorsal-to-plantar (Fig. 3D). This elevates the soft tissue from the medial, dorsal, and lateral aspects of the metatarsal surgical neck. An incision through the periosteum in line with the long axis of the metatarsal also can be performed, followed by elevation of the periosteum off of the underlying metatarsal. The senior author (TSR) does not perform this maneuver unless it is necessary to resect a segment of bone to create shortening of the metatarsal [23]. Under intraoperative image intensification control, a narrow-width (5 mm), medium-length power saw is used to create an osteotomy from dorsal-to-plantar, angulated slightly proximal-to-distal to allow for simultaneous dorsal and proximal translation of the capital fragment (Fig. 3E, F). Following use of the saw blade, a small osteotome is inserted into the osteotomy site, and the metatarsal head is pried distally in order verify completion of the osteotomy. Another useful maneuver is to perform the same thumb-to-index finger maneuver described previously, followed by repeated dorsal-to-plantar translation of the metatarsal head to verify completion release of any soft-tissue or osseous structures that otherwise would limit the mobility of the osteotomy. No internal fixation is employed, as the metatarsal head is bound through the deep transverse intermetatarsal ligaments and dense capsule–ligamentous structures about the metatarsophalangeal joint, limiting catastrophic displacement when performed correctly. Additionally, it should be understood that the intention of this osteotomy is to allow the metatarsal head to "seek its own level" (Fig. 3G). The surgical site then is irrigated, and the skin is closed with a single 2-0 nylon in vertical mattress fashion and metallic skin staples. A bulky, well-padded dressing from toes-to-knee as described previously [47] is applied with extra padding directly underneath and osteotomized metatarsal head to maintain dorsal translation. The patient is allowed to perform partial weight bearing in the same postoperative shoe and orthosis system described previously with a gait aide. The initial surgical dressings are removed in 5 to 7 days unless a wound is present that requires closer monitoring, and then every 7 to 10 days thereafter if necessary. When performed correctly, the osteotomy will develop rapid osseous callus formation (Fig. 3H), followed by maturation and remodeling over time (Fig. 3I). The senior author (TSR) restricts the use of this osteotomy to high-risk patients who have plantar ulcerative lesions recalcitrant to conservative wound-healing modalities or recurrent despite these treatments to surgically off-load the deformity by decreasing the plantar pressure associated with the metatarsal deformity [43,67]. In the senior author's experience (TSR), it is a universal finding that the ulceration heals within 10 to 14 days following the osteotomy, because the underlying deformity has been corrected (Fig. 3J). Once fully healed, the patient is placed into an extra-depth shoe with accommodative multidensity orthoses for life.

White [22] conducted a limited retrospective review of 62 second metatarsal, 29 third metatarsal, and 17 fourth metatarsal minimal incision unfixated osteotomies and reported two delayed unions (0.3%), one (0.2%) malunion, and no nonunions for the second metatarsal osteotomies performed. The delayed unions were attributed to improper placement of the osteotomy distal to the metaphyseal–diaphyseal junction at the metatarsal head–neck junction, thereby disrupting the vascular supply to the metatarsal head as discussed previously. Except for the very specific indications discussed by the authors in this article, because of the paucity of peer-reviewed published literature, the routine use of minimal-incision osteotomies about the central metatarsals in patients not considered at high risk should be performed with caution.

Fifth metatarsal vascular supply

The extraosseous vascular supply to the fifth metatarsal occurs by means of three main vessels, similar to the supply of the first metatarsal:

1. The dorsal metatarsal artery, arising from the arcuate artery, the lateral tarsal artery, or the proximal perforating artery of the fourth interspace
2. The plantar metatarsal artery arising from the lateral plantar artery
3. An inconsistent branch of the lateral plantar artery [66,68].

The dorsal metatarsal artery travels distally in the intermetatarsal space dorsal to the dorsal interosseous muscle. The plantar metatarsal artery supplies the plantar aspect of the fifth metatarsal by forming a union with the deep plantar branch of the dorsalis pedis artery. The plantar arch supplies a superficial metatarsal artery running plantar to the interossei along the midline of the shaft, and a deep plantar metatarsal artery also may be present coursing between the plantar and dorsal interossei. Most of the extraosseous supply of the fifth metatarsal courses along its medial aspect. The intraosseous vascular supply to the fifth metatarsal consists of: the periosteal plexus; a single-nutrient artery, entering at the medial cortical junction of the proximal and middle third of the metatarsal shaft; and the metaphyseal–epiphyseal vessels that are intracapsular [66,68].

Minimum-incision fifth metatarsal osteotomy: surgical technique

The surgical technique begins as described previously for minimum-incision first and central metatarsal osteotomies. Following the thumb-to-index finger maneuver described previously, a 1 cm vertical incision is placed through the skin overlying the dorsal–lateral aspect of the fifth metatarsal. A hemostat with the jaws fully closed then is used to dissect down to the level of the capsule and periosteum. Once the bone is palpated, the hemostat jaws are opened, with one jaw placed dorsal and the other plantar until the hemostat can be advanced from lateral-to-medial. This elevates the soft tissue from the lateral, dorsal, and plantar aspect of the fifth metatarsal and is the same technique described previously for performing minimum incision osteotomy of the first and central metatarsals. A 1.6 mm Steinmann pin is inserted at the lateral aspect of the fifth toe plantar to the lateral nail border and advanced proximally along the lateral aspect of the fifth toe phalanges to the level of the metatarsophalangeal joint. At this point, the fifth toe is placed into an overcorrected position, and the Steinmann pin is advanced along the lateral border of the fifth metatarsal head until visualized at the distal edge of the skin incision. Under intraoperative image intensification control, a narrow-width (5 mm), medium-length power saw is used to create an osteotomy from lateral-to-medial, angulated slightly proximal-to-distal to allow for simultaneous medial and dorsal translation of the capital fragment. Following use of the saw blade, a small osteotome is inserted into the osteotomy site and the metatarsal head is pried distally in order to verify completion of the osteotomy. Another useful maneuver is to perform the same thumb-to-index finger maneuver described previously, followed by repeated dorsal-to-plantar translation of the metatarsal head to verify completion release of any soft-tissue or osseous structures that otherwise would limit the mobility of the osteotomy. Under image intensification, the fifth toe and metatarsal head then are maneuvered medially using the Steinmann pin as a toggle, while the fifth metatarsal shaft is distracted laterally with a small elevator inserted into the medullary canal. Once proper alignment is verified, the Steinmann pin is advanced into the medullary canal of the fifth metatarsal until it contacts the base of the fifth metatarsal. This process is essentially a mirror image of the technique employed for the minimum-incision first metatarsal osteotomy described previously. The surgical site then is irrigated, and the skin is closed with a single 2-0 nylon in vertical mattress fashion and metallic skin staples. A bulky, well-padded dressing from toes-to-knee [47] is applied as discussed previously. The initial surgical dressings are removed in 5 to 7 days unless a wound is present that requires closer monitoring, and then every 7 to 10 days thereafter. The patient is allowed partial weight bearing with a gait aide but strictly prohibited from rolling-off of the forefoot for 6 to 8 weeks or until there is evidence of osseous callus formation about the osteotomy site. Once this occurs, the Steinman pin is removed in the office under aseptic technique and guarded full weight bearing is initiated using the same postoperative shoe and orthosis system mentioned previously [47]. As with minimum-incision central metatarsal osteotomies, the senior author (TSR) restricts the use of this osteotomy to high-risk patients who have plantar or plantar–lateral ulcerative lesions recalcitrant to conservative wound healing modalities or recurrent despite these treatments to surgically off-load the deformity by decreasing the plantar pressure associated with the metatarsal deformity [43,67]. Once fully healed, the patient is placed into an extradepth shoe with accommodative multidensity orthoses for life.

White [22] performed a limited retrospective review of 40 fifth metatarsal minimal incision unfixated osteotomies and reported two nonunions (5%), one mal-union (3%), and no delayed unions. Catanzariti and colleagues [69] performed a retrospective review of 38 open unfixated fifth metatarsal osteotomies performed similar to the technique reported previously and reported 14 (35%) transfer lesions, 10 (26%) recurrent deformities, and no nonunions. Because of these findings, the authors concluded that the routine use of open, unfixated fifth metatarsal osteotomies should not be performed because of the significant incidence of sagittal plane malalignment and associated development of transfer lesions [69].Other authors, however, performed a similar retrospective review of 50 open, unfixated fifth metatarsal osteotomies found no nonunions and a mean dorsal displacement of 3 mm with a mean shortening of 2 mm. There was no mention of the incidence of lesion recurrence or transfer metatarsalgia [70]. A retrospective review compared fixated and un-fixated distal fifth metatarsal osteotomy of varying configurations with most being similar osteotomy configuration to the procedure described previously [71] but performed in traditional open fashion. The unfixated group had a significantly increased incidence of dorsal displacement (mean: 2 mm) and shortening (mean: 2.7 mm) compared with the fixated group. These authors concluded that the use of internal fixation provides a more predictable healing pattern, degree of correction, and less dorsal displacement and shortening than un-fixated fifth metatarsal osteotomies [71]. Weitzel and colleagues [25] conducted a retrospective review of 30 fifth metatarsal osteotomies performed in open fashion but with a similar osteotomy configuration and intramedullary Steinmann pin fixation as described in this article with a mean of follow-up of 7 years and 8 months. The authors reported three pin site infections (10%), two recurrent deformities (6.7%), one (3.3%) incidence of transfer metatarsalgia, and one (3.3%) delayed union. Legenstein and colleagues [26] performed a retrospective review of 77 feet treated with the Bösch technique applied to the fifth metatarsal including the intramedullary Steinmann pin fixation with a mean follow-up of 56.6 months. The authors reported four (5.2%) infections, one (1.3%) incidence of transfer metatarsal metatarsalgia, and no nonunions. Martinelli and Valentini [27] performed a limited retrospective review of 25 fifth metatarsal minimal-incision fixated osteotomies as described by Weitzel and colleagues [25] in 20 patients and reported one (4%) hypertrophic nonunion, one (4%) malunion, and one (4%) superficial infection. Giannini and colleagues [72] performed a limited retrospective review of 50 fifth metatarsal minimal-incision fixated osteotomies similar to the first metatarsal osteotomy described by Giannini and colleagues [10] in 32 patients and reported one (2%) superficial infection and two (4%) transfer lesions to the fourth metatarsal. When reviewing the previously mentioned literature, it becomes clear that the osteotomy configuration discussed here is effective at correcting the underlying fifth metatarsal deformity and that the use of internal fixation reduces the incidence of malunion.

Summary

This article focused on minimal-incision metatarsal osteotomies for treating ulcerative lesions related to hallux valgus deformities and central or fifth metatarsal plantar ulcerations to correct the structural deformity responsible for the ulceration. Advantages of minimum-incision techniques, especially when applied to the high-risk patient and when performed by surgeons experienced with these techniques, are that they result in less soft-tissue and osseous trauma, specifically preservation of the vascular supply to these tissues, reduce operating time, and result in less postoperative bleeding. The limited disruption of soft-tissue attachments also maintains the intrinsic osseous stability following central metatarsal osteotomy. First and fifth metatarsal osteotomies, however, are more predictable when an inexpensive Steinmann pin is used as described for internal fixation. A review of the literature regarding the minimum-incision surgical techniques available for the first, central, and fifth metatarsals has been presented in detail. Although a steep learning curve exists with these procedures, the advantage of their use in high-risk populations, when combined with proper protected postoperative ambulation and life-long use of appropriate shoe-gear, will resolve a recalcitrant or recurrent neuropathic ulceration rapidly and predictably by correcting the underlying structural deformity with minimal complications.

References

[1] Van Enoo RE, Cane EM. Minimal incision surgery: a plastic technique or a cover-up? Clin Podiatr Med Surg 1986;3(2):321–35.
[2] Hymes L. Introduction: brief history of the use of minimum incision surgery (MIS). In: Fielding MD, editor. Forefoot minimum incision in podiatric medicine: a handbook on primary corrective procedures on the human foot using minimum incisions with minimum trauma. New York: Futura Pub Co; 1977. p. 1–2.
[3] David C, Sammarco G, James G. Minimum incision surgery. Foot Ankle Int 1992;13(3): 157–60.

[4] Gorecki GA, Weissman S, Kidawa AS. Lixiscope: a podiatric evaluation. J Am Podiatry Assoc 1982;72(6):304–9.
[5] Bösch P, Wanke S, Legenstein R. Hallux valgus correction by the method of Bösch: a new technique with a seven-to-ten-year follow-up. Foot Ankle Clin 2000;5(3):485–98.
[6] Hohmann G. Symptomatische oder phisiologische Behandlung des Hallux valgus. Münch Med Wochenschr 1921;68(2):1042–5.
[7] Lamprecht E, Kramer J. Die Metatarsale-I-Osteotomie nach Behandlung des Hallux valgus. Orthopaedische Praxis 1982;8(5):636–45.
[8] Roven MD. Ambulatory correction of hallux abducto valgus: angulational, transpositional, derotation, and hallux set procedure. Clin Podiatry 1985;2(3):503–9.
[9] Weinberger BH, Fulp JM, Falstrom P, et al. Retrospective evaluation of percutaneous bunionectomies and distal osteotomies without internal fixation. Clin Podiatr Med Surg 1991;8(1):111–36.
[10] Giannini S, Ceccarelli F, Bevoni R, et al. Hallux valgus surgery: the minimally invasive bunion correction (SERI). Techniques in Foot and Ankle Surgery 2003;2(1):11–20.
[11] Chomiak J. [Initial experience with subcapital osteotomy of the first metatarsus for hallux valgus by the closed method]. Acta Chir Orthop Traumatol Cech 1991;58(3):157–66 [in Czech].
[12] Portaluri M. Hallux valgus correction by the method of Bösch: a clinical evaluation. Foot Ankle Clin 2000;5(3):499–511.
[13] López JJG, Rodríguez SR, Méndez LC. Functional, esthetic, and radiographic results of treatment of hallux valgus with minimally invasive surgery. Acta Orthopedica Mexicana 2005;19(Suppl 1):S42–6.
[14] Sanna P, Ruiu GA. Percutaneous distal osteotomy of the first metatarsal (PDO) for the surgical treatment of hallux valgus. Chir Organi Mov 2005;90(4):365–9.
[15] Magnan B, Pezzé L, Rossi N, et al. Percutaneous distal metatarsal osteotomy for correction of hallux valgus. J Bone Joint Surg Am 2005;87(6):1191–9.
[16] Magnan B, Bortolazzi R, Samaila E, et al. Percutaneous distal metatarsal osteotomy for correction of hallux valgus: surgical technique. J Bone Joint Surg Am 2006;88(Suppl 1): S135–48.
[17] Migues A, Campaner G, Slullitel G, et al. Minimally invasive surgery in hallux valgus and digital deformities. Orthopedics 2007;30(7):523–8.
[18] DiMarcantonio T. MIS bunion correction offers advantages over open technique, but questions remain. Techniques in Foot and Ankle Surgery 2007;10(5):13–6.
[19] DiMarcantonio T. SERI osteotomy yields more complications than Scarf and Akin for bunion deformity. Orthopaedics Today International 2007;10(9):18–20.
[20] Kadakia AR, Smerek JP, Myerson MS. Radiographic results after percutaneous distal metatarsal osteotomy for correction of hallux valgus deformity. Foot Ankle Int 2007;28(3):355–60.
[21] Hymes L. Bone procedure: lesser metatarsals. In: Fielding MD, editor. Forefoot minimum incision in podiatric medicine: a handbook on primary corrective procedures on the human foot using minimum incisions with minimum trauma. New York: Futura Pub Co; 1977. p. 147–74.
[22] White DL. Minimal-incision approach to osteotomies of the lesser metatarsals for treatment of intractable keratosis, metatarsalgia, and Tailor's bunion. Clin Podiatr Med Surg 1991; 8(1):25–39.
[23] Roukis TS. Central metatarsal head–neck osteotomies: indications and operative techniques. Clin Podiatr Med Surg 2005;22(2):197–222.
[24] Roukis TS. The Tailor's bunionette deformity: a field guide to surgical correction. Clin Podiatr Med Surg 2005;22(2):223–45.
[25] Weitzel S, Trnka H-J, Petroutsas J. Transverse medial slide osteotomy for bunionette deformity: long-term results. Foot Ankle Int 2007;28(7):794–8.
[26] Legenstein R, Bonomo J, Huber W, et al. Correction of Tailor's bunion with the Bösch technique: a retrospective study. Foot Ankle Int 2007;28(7):799–803.

[27] Martinelli B, Valentini R. Correction of valgus of the fifth metatarsal and varus of the fifth toe by percutaneous distal osteotomy. Foot and Ankle Surgery 2007;13(3):136–9.

[28] Panchbhavi VK. Technique tip: buttress Kirschner wire fixation for distal chevron osteotomy. Foot Ankle Int 2007;28(11):133–4.

[29] Wu DY. Syndesmosis procedure. A nonosteotomy approach to metatarsus primus varus correction. Foot Ankle Int 2007;28(9):1000–6.

[30] Holmes BG Jr. Correction of hallux valgus deformity using the mini tightrope device. Techniques in Foot and Ankle Surgery 2008;7(1):9–16.

[31] Young MJ, Cavanagh PR, Thomas G, et al. The effect of callus removal on dynamic plantar foot pressures in diabetic patients. Diabet Med 1992;9(8):55–7.

[32] Fleischli JG, Lavery LA, Vela SA, et al. Comparison of strategies for reducing pressure at the site of neuropathic ulcers. J Am Podiatr Med Assoc 1997;87(10):466–72.

[33] Armstrong DG, Peters EJ, Athanasiou KA, et al. Is there a critical level of plantar foot pressure to identify patients at risk for neuropathic foot ulceration? J Foot Ankle Surg 1998;37(4):303–7.

[34] Armstrong DG, Nguyen HC, Lavry LA, et al. Off-loading the diabetic foot wound: a randomized clinical trial. Diabetes Care 2001;24(6):1019–22.

[35] Birke JA, Fred B, Krieger LA, et al. The effectiveness of an accommodative dressing in offloading pressure over areas of previous metatarsal head ulceration. Wounds 2003;15(2):33–9.

[36] Mueller MJ, Lott DJ, Hastings MK, et al. Efficacy and mechanism of orthotic devices to unload metatarsal heads in people with diabetes and history of plantar ulcers. Phys Ther 2006;86(6):833–42.

[37] Hastings MK, Mueller MJ, Pilgram TK, et al. Effect of metatarsal pad placement on plantar pressure in people with diabetes mellitus and peripheral neuropathy. Foot Ankle Int 2007;28(1):84–8.

[38] Armstrong DG, Lavery LA, Bushman TR. Peak foot pressures influence the healing time of diabetic foot ulcers treated with total contact casts. J Rehabil Res Dev 1998;35(1):1–5.

[39] Sinacore DR. Healing times of diabetic ulcers in the presence of fixed deformities of the foot using total contact casting. Foot Ankle Int 1998;19(9):613–8.

[40] Mantey I, Foster AV, Spencer S, et al. Why do foot ulcers recur in diabetic patients? Diabet Med 1999;16(3):245–9.

[41] Boyko EJ, Ahroni JH, Stensel V, et al. A prospective study of risk factors for diabetic foot ulcers: the Seattle diabetic foot study. Diabetes Care 1999;22(7):1036–42.

[42] Reiber GE, Smith DG, Wallace C, et al. Effect of therapeutic footwear on reulceration in patients with diabetes: a randomized controlled trial. J Am Med Assoc 2002;287(19):2552–8.

[43] Frigg A, Pagenstert G, Schäfer D, et al. Recurrence and prevention of diabetic foot ulcers after total contact casting. Foot Ankle Int 2007;28(1):64–9.

[44] Shereff MJ, Yang QM, Kummer FJ. Extraosseous and intraosseous arterial supply to the first metatarsal and metatarsophalangeal joint. Foot Ankle 1987;8(2):81–93.

[45] Piqué-Vidal C. The effect of temperature elevation during discontinuous use of rotatory burrs in the correction of hallux valgus. J Foot Ankle Surg 2005;44(5):336–44.

[46] Barouk LS. Scarf osteotomy for hallux valgus correction: local anatomy, surgical technique, and combination with other forefoot procedures. Foot Ankle Clin 2000;5(3):525–58.

[47] Andersen CA, Roukis TS. The diabetic foot. Surg Clin North Am 2007;87(5):1149–77.

[48] Viladot R, Alvarado OJ, Arancibia M, et al. Hallux valgus: a modified Kramer osteotomy. Foot Ankle Surg 2007;13(3):126–31.

[49] Jones KJ, Feiwell LA, Freedman EL, et al. The effect of chevron osteotomy with lateral capsular release on the blood supply to the first metatarsal head. J Bone Joint Surg Am 1995;77(2):197–204.

[50] Malal JJ, Shaw-Dunn J, Kumar CS. Blood supply to the first metatarsal head and vessels at risk with a chevron osteotomy. J Bone Joint Surg Am 2007;89(9):2018–22.

[51] Kuhn MA, Lippert FG, Phipps MJ, et al. Blood flow to the metatarsal head after chevron osteotomy. Foot Ankle Int 2005;26(7):526–9.

[52] Neary MT, Jones RO, Sunshein K, et al. Avascular necrosis of the first metatarsal head following Austin osteotomy: a follow-up study. J Foot Ankle Surg 1993;32(5):503–35.

[53] Green MA, Dorris MF, Baessler TP, et al. Avascular necrosis following distal chevron osteotomy of the first metatarsal. J Foot Ankle Surg 1993;32(6):617–22.

[54] Peterson DA, Ziberfarb JL, Greene MA, et al. Avascular necrosis of the first metatarsal head: incidence in distal osteotomy combined with lateral soft-tissue release. Foot Ankle 1994;15(2):59–63.

[55] Schuberth JM, Reilly CH, Gudas CJ. The closing wedge osteotomy: a critical analysis of first metatarsal elevation. J Am Podiatry Assoc 1984;74(1):13–24.

[56] Kummer FJ. Mathematical analysis of first metatarsal osteotomies. Foot Ankle 1989;9(6): 281–9.

[57] Roukis TS, Scherer PR, Anderson CF. Position of the first ray and motion of the first metatarsophalangeal joint. J Am Podiatr Med Assoc 1996;86(11):538–46.

[58] Cicchinelli LD, Camasta CA, McGlamry ED. Iatrogenic metatarsus primus elevatus: etiology, evaluation, and surgical management. J Am Podiatr Med Assoc 1997;87(4):165–77.

[59] Roukis TS. Metatarsus primus elevatus in hallux rigidus: fact or fiction? J Am Podiatr Med Assoc 2005;95(3):221–8.

[60] Roukis TS, Zgonis T. A compendium of personal experience with complications of first ray surgery. The Journal of Foot Surgery (India) 2005;20(2):111–39.

[61] Dhukaram V, Hullin MG, Kumar CS. The Mitchell and Scarf osteotomies for hallux valgus correction: a retrospective, comparative analysis using plantar pressures. J Foot Ankle Surg 2006;45(6):400–9.

[62] Tóth K, Huszanyik I, Kellermann P, et al. The effect of first ray shortening in the development of metatarsalgia in the second through fourth rays after metatarsal osteotomy. Foot Ankle Int 2007;28(1):61–3.

[63] Yíldírím Y, Saygí B, Aydín N, et al. Components of the Wilson osteotomy that are effective on hallux valgus repair. J Foot Ankle Surg 2007;46(1):21–6.

[64] Saro C, Andrén B, Wildemyr Z, et al. Outcome after distal metatarsal osteotomy for hallux valgus: a prospective randomized controlled trial of two methods. Foot Ankle Int 2007; 28(7):778–87.

[65] Peterson WJ, Lankes JM, Paulsen F, et al. The arterial supply of the lesser metatarsal heads: a vascular injection study in human cadavers. Foot Ankle Int 2002;23(6):491–5.

[66] Shereff MJ, Yang QM, Kummer FJ, et al. Vascular anatomy of the fifth metatarsal. Foot Ankle 1991;11(6):350–3.

[67] Khalafi A, Landsman AS, Lautenschlager EP, et al. Plantar forefoot pressure changes after second metatarsal neck osteotomy. Foot Ankle Int 2005;26(7):1–6.

[68] Smith JW, Amoczky SP, Hersh A. The intraosseous blood supply of the fifth metatarsal: implications for proximal fracture healing. Foot Ankle 1992;13(3):143–52.

[69] Catanzariti AR, Friedman C, DiStazio J. Oblique osteotomy of the fifth metatarsal: a five-year review. J Foot Surg 1988;27(4):316–20.

[70] Zvijac JE, Janecki CJ, Freeling RM. Distal oblique osteotomy for tailor's bunion. Foot Ankle 1991;12(3):171–5.

[71] Pontious J, Brook JW, Hillstrom HJ. Tailor's bunion: is fixation necessary? J Am Podiatr Med Assoc 1996;86(2):63–73.

[72] Giannini S, Faldini C, Vannini F, et al. The minimally invasive osteotomy SERI (simple, effective, rapid, inexpensive) for correction of bunionette deformity. Foot Ankle Int 2008; 29(3):282–6.

ELSEVIER
SAUNDERS

Clin Podiatr Med Surg
25 (2008) 609–622

CLINICS IN
PODIATRIC
MEDICINE AND
SURGERY

Minimum-Incision Ray Resection

Ali Öznur, MD[a],
Thomas S. Roukis, DPM, FACFAS[b],*

[a]Department of Orthopaedics and Traumatology,
Hacettepe University, Sihhiye 06100, Ankara, Turkey
[b]Limb Preservation Service, Vascular/Endovascular Surgery Service,
Department of Surgery, Madigan Army Medical Center,
9040-A Fitzsimmons Avenue, MCHJ-SV, Tacoma, WA 98431, USA

Diabetic forefoot ulcerations are a common pedal manifestation and have a multitude of etiologies. The presence of dense peripheral neuropathy [1], pedal deformity (ie, intrinsic minus foot type) [1–3], limited joint mobility [4–6], equinus contracture of the posterior calf musculature [7–10], distal displacement or atrophy of the plantar forefoot padding [1–6], and peripheral arterial disease [1,11,12], however, usually coexist. These processes make the goal of eradicating infection, providing stable wound closure, and restoring a stable plantigrade, shoeable/braceable foot a significant challenge [1]. Treatment of the infected plantar forefoot ulceration, especially about the central metatarsals, creates a particularly difficult challenge because of the specialized nature of the soft tissues, relatively limited soft-tissue coverage options, and significant shear and tangential forces sustained during stance and the gait cycle [13–15].

Indications for a ray resection include localized gangrene of the toe and web spaces, infection of the toe with extension into the metatarsophalangeal joint or intermetatarsal spaces because of contiguous spread, or osteomyelitis of a toe and/or metatarsal head [16–21]. Each of these scenarios creates a situation where amputation of the toe alone will not allow for adequate soft-tissue coverage of the resultant defect, thereby leaving the metatarsal exposed and avascular. Performing a metatarsal resection in conjunction with the toe amputation allows for sufficient soft-tissue coverage of the

The opinions or assertions contained herein are the private view of the author and are not to be construed as official or reflecting the views of the Department of the Army or the Department of Defense.
* Corresponding author.
E-mail address: thomas.s.roukis@us.army.mil (T.S. Roukis).

0891-8422/08/$ - see front matter. Published by Elsevier Inc.
doi:10.1016/j.cpm.2008.05.008

toe amputation site and, when performed properly, leaves a balanced, functional, albeit slightly narrower forefoot that can be fitted properly into protective shoe gear and accommodative insoles [16–21]. In practice, isolated ray resection of one of the three central rays is technically more difficult than performing border (ie, first and fifth metatarsal) ray resections. In certain instances, two adjacent metatarsal ray resections can be performed with the same end result. This is especially true for the second and third and fourth and fifth combined ray resections, which tend to be quite functional. The natural history of great toe amputations, however, and first ray resections [22,23], as well as three or more toe amputations or three or more ray resections [24–33] do not support the use of these procedures as definitive procedures in high-risk patients, especially those who have concomitant foot and lower extremity deformities, sensory–motor neuropathy, and peripheral vascular disease. If these procedures are necessary in this patient population, it is the authors' opinion that strong consideration should be given to performing a well-balanced transmetatarsal amputation [34–36] or internal pedal amputation [37].

The traditional approaches to central metatarsal head ulcerations have involved either limited osseous resection, with or without amputation of the associated toe [11,12,16,17], or resection of the entire metatarsal [18–21]. In the traditional ray resection technique, a tennis-racquet incision is made circumferentially around the base of the toe, with a single limb extending proximally over the dorsum of the involved metatarsal. Unfortunately, the proximal extension of the incision may jeopardize future incisions necessary to perform more proximal amputations if the ray resection procedure fails. Additionally, it disrupts the fragile vasculature that courses within the intermetatarsal spaces and intrinsic musculature, thereby increasing the risk of wound dehiscence and subsequent infection [11]. Finally, the traditional approach to ray resection creates a cleft-foot deformity that is prone to transfer ulceration and recurrent wound breakdown because of the unstable nature of the forefoot [38].

To expedite healing and create a stable, plantigrade forefoot following central metatarsal ray resection, narrowing of the forefoot through manual apposition of the medial and lateral forefoot segments has been advocated using widely spaced, heavy- gauge sutures and splint immobilization to provide stability until soft-tissue healing has occurred [16–19]. Although this concept inherently makes sense, the clinical application of this technique has a large inherent flaw, that being relying on the tension across the adjacent soft tissues and external support to provide soft-tissue and skeletal stability in already compromised tissues.

With this concept in mind, Hansen [39] described resection of the entire ray, including a segment of the adjacent cuneiform or cuboid, which allows the adjacent metatarsals to become approximated and obliterates any dead space formation. He described the use of compression internal fixation using at least one screw across the cuneiforms and/or cuboid and another across the metatarsals to stabilize the narrowed forefoot similar in concept to a technique described previously by Smith [20]. Although sound in theory, this technique is difficult to perform in practice because of the relative osteopenia present in patients who have diabetes [1,40]. Additionally, it requires prolonged nonweight-bearing immobilization and carries with it the inherent risk of deep infection about the retained hardware, hardware failure or prominence, and development of nonunion or malunion about the cuneiform and/or cuboid osteotomy site(s).

Strauss and colleagues [41] employed the same concept proposed by Hansen [39] and Smith [20] but employed the use of manual apposition of the forefoot, insertion of a series of half-pins in the first and fifth metatarsals, which were connected to a triangular or cathedral-like external fixation system. The authors discussed exploiting the viscoelastic properties of the forefoot soft tissues and articulations [42] through repeated manual compression of the forefoot and locking-unlocking-locking the external fixation system over a 5- to 10-minute period to completely obliterate the dead space cleft. Subsequent dorsal and/or plantar soft-tissue defects were closed in primary fashion, left to heal by means of secondary intent over time, or covered with a split-thickness skin graft. The authors described the concomitant use of hyperbaric oxygen in 14 of their 15 patients in addition to prolonged nonweight-bearing immobilization. Careful analysis of the data presented reveals a significant number of patient compliance issues as would be expected with a bulky, heavy, external fixation device that mandates nonweight-bearing immobilization and frequent office visits for local wound care and hyperbaric oxygen treatments. Additionally, the need to use prolonged intraoperative manual compression and manipulation of the external fixation device to achieve complete closure of the cleft foot deformity represents a disadvantage of this specific form of external fixation, especially when taking into account the cost of operating room time required to assemble the device and repeatedly manipulate it. The concept of employing an external fixation device to stabilize cleft foot deformities, however, proved sound in that of the 12 (87%) patients who resumed ambulation, a mechanically sound forefoot remained that was cosmetically appealing to the patients and readily shoeable/braceable [41].

Öznur and Tokgözoğlu [43] employed the same inherent concept of Strauss and colleagues [41] but employed the use of two external fixation system half-rings and dueling medial and lateral olive wires that were tensioned after creating an osteotomy at the level of the base of the remaining lateral metatarsals. Through graduated tension across the opposing olive wires, gradual and precise closure of the cleft deformity was performed. The patients were allowed limited weight sharing during the time the external fixation device was employed [44,45].

Bernstein and Guerin [46] presented the use of a mini-external fixator originally intended for bone lengthening and transport to achieve gradual closure of the resultant forefoot defect following central ray resection.

The closure occurred over a 30-day period, which was followed by removal of the device and application of a total contact cast for 2 weeks. Bibbo [47] employed a similar technique but achieved complete wound closure in the operating room along with primary closure of the dorsal incision used to perform central ray resection, which replaced his prior technique of serial tightening of transosseous metatarsal wires with local wound care and eventual coverage with a split-thickness skin graft.

Most recently, Zgonis and colleagues [38] discussed the use of a split-thickness skin graft within the cleft space followed by use of a circular external ring fixator that allowed:

Precise narrowing of the forefoot without the need for osteotomy of the metatarsals or their tarsal components
Weight sharing during the postoperative recovery period
Limited duration of external fixation use
Rapid healing by means of application of a split-thickness skin graft about the remaining cleft foot deformity, which has the added benefit of producing additional scarring and contracture over time during the skin graft maturation process

Although the use of external fixation to close the problematic cleft foot deformity represents a major advancement over previous techniques, the prolonged time required to afford complete wound closure represents a significant disadvantage, because it is accepted that the longer a wound remains open, the greater the likelihood of developing an infection [1,48,49]. Additionally, the fairly short time frame that a patient will tolerate the presence of an external fixation device attached to his or her foot and lower limb is an important consideration [50]. With these concepts in mind, the authors have used a minimum-incision technique [51] to decrease the dorsal soft-tissue dissection necessary to expose the metatarsal without compromising the resection, which maintains an intact soft-tissue envelope and preserves vascularity within the intermetatarsal spaces. This approach has the added benefit of allowing direct primary closure of the incisions in most patients. If necessary, a mini-external fixator device or half-ring system can be applied to rapidly approximate the skin edges in patients who have decreased compliance of their skin, as seen in long-standing uncontrolled diabetes [4–7] or nonreconstructable peripheral vascular disease where tension about the incision sites will lead to necrosis [12,18,25].

Minimum-incision ray resection

The surgical procedure begins with the patient positioned in the supine position on the operating room table with a well-padded bolster placed beneath the ipsilateral buttock to control physiologic external rotation of the lower limb. The procedure most commonly is performed under local regional anesthesia (ie, ankle or popliteal block) and monitored sedation.

A contraindication to use of local regional anesthesia is the presence of active infection or gangrene in the field intended to be infiltrated. The use of a tourniquet is not necessary because of the limited soft-tissue dissection afforded by this procedure, and it is contraindicated in the high-risk patient. The initial debridement must be radical and include all obvious nonviable soft tissue to establish a viable, healthy, and well-perfused wound bed [52–55]. If this cannot be achieved with the proposed minimal incision ray resection, then either the traditional approach should be chosen or definitive treatment delayed until delayed primary closure with or without additional soft-tissue coverage techniques is deemed appropriate [52–55].

The involved toe should be grasped with a towel clamp through the distal interphalangeal joint (Fig. 1A) to facilitate dissection by employing the clamp as a toggle to move the toe and limit handling of the infected, necrotic tissue by the surgical team, which maintains an aseptic surgical field. Converging semielliptic incisions are placed about the base of the toe at the level of the midshaft of the proximal phalanx and carried directly to bone. A small periosteal elevator is used to elevate the soft tissues off of the shaft and base of the proximal phalanx to expose the metatarsophalangeal joint, which then is incised circumferentially to amputate the toe. The capsule to the metatarsophalangeal joint is freed from the dorsal, medial, and lateral aspects of the metatarsal with a No. 10 blade to the metaphyseal–diaphyseal junction. Next, a small periosteal elevator is inserted in subperiosteal fashion and advanced proximally along the shaft of the metatarsal to the proximal metaphyseal–diaphyseal junction (Fig. 1B) that is verified under intraoperative image intensification. The periosteal elevator is withdrawn from the surgical site and then advanced along the medial and lateral aspects of the metatarsal in subperiosteal fashion as described for the dorsal aspect. Finally, a small, curved metatarsal scoop-type elevator is placed plantarly between the metatarsal head and plantar plate and advanced proximally in subperiosteal fashion as described. This effectively shells-out the metatarsal while preserving the vasculature to the intrinsic musculature. Once the metatarsal has been freed, the proximal extent of subperiosteal dissection on the involved metatarsal is identified under image intensification (Fig. 1C), and a 1 cm transverse incision is marked at this location. The incision is carried through the skin only and is followed by blunt dissection with a hemostat in line with the incision to the underlying metatarsal, with care taken to mobilize any regional soft-tissue structures out of the surgical field. The jaws of the hemostat then are opened, and the hemostat is advanced to define the medial and lateral borders of the metatarsal (Fig. 1D). This also serves to elevate the intrinsic musculature off of the respective aspects of the involved metatarsal, thereby protecting the regional vascular anatomy. Care is taken not to inadvertently create an osteotomy in an uninvolved metatarsal. Under direct image intensification, a narrow-width (ie, 5 mm), long-length saw blade is passed from dorsal-to-plantar at the level of the proximal metaphyseal–diaphyseal junction (Fig. 1E).

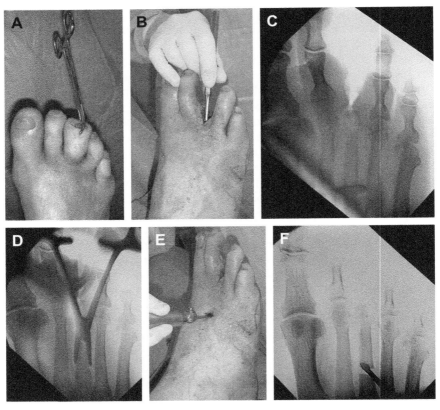

Fig. 1. Intraoperative photograph demonstrating the use of a sharp towel clamp placed dorsal-to-plantar through the distal interphalangeal joint of the third toe for control of the toe during dissection and to employ no-touch technique (*A*). A periosteal elevator is shown being advanced across the dorsal aspect of the third metatarsal in subperiosteal fashion (*B*) until it reaches the proximal metaphyseal–diaphyseal junction as verified under intraoperative image intensification with the use of a metallic instrument (*C*). A hemostat is used to free the intrinsic musculature off of the metatarsal and verify the proper location and metatarsal before osteotomy (*D*). A narrow-width, long-length saw blade is used to complete the osteotomy (*E*) followed by insertion of a small osteotome or periosteal elevator to pry the transected metatarsal distally, verifying complete transection and release of the surrounding soft tissues (*F*). The metatarsal head then is grasped through the distal incision, and the metatarsal is retrieved in toto (*G*). Adherence to the technique described allows for atraumatic amputation of the toe (*left*) and a skeletonized metatarsal free of soft-tissue (*right*) (*H*). Intraoperative image intensification view of the forefoot following minimum incision ray resection before (*I*) and following manual compression of the forefoot (*J*), revealing easy closure of the soft-tissue defect without tension (*K*). Note the presence of a suction drain that has been sutured distally and stapled proximally at the exit site from the incision used to perform the metatarsal osteotomy.

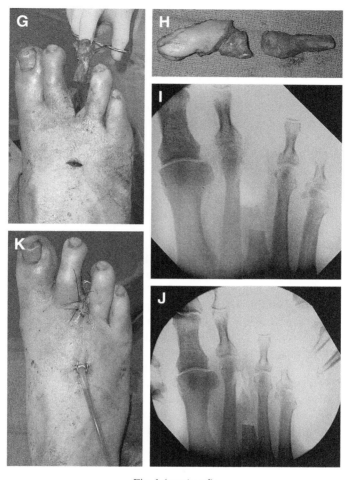

Fig. 1 (*continued*)

Alternatively, a 1.5 mm drill can be employed to make several drill holes over the osteotomy level, which then are connected with an osteotome and mallet. Once the osteotomy has been completed, a small osteotome is introduced into the osteotomy, and the metatarsal is levered distally to verify complete release from any soft tissue restraints (Fig. 1F). The metatarsal head then is grasped through the toe amputation incision with a clamp and retrieved from the foot (Fig. 1G). By performing the technique as described previously, amputation of the toe and resection of the metatarsal can be performed in en block fashion rather than piecemeal (Fig. 1H). The fifth metatarsal should be osteotomized obliquely from dorsal-distal-lateral to plantar-proximal-medial. The proximal part of the shaft is left to enhance the weight-bearing area and retain the insertion of peroneus brevis tendon.

The forefoot is compressed manually from medial-to-lateral (Fig. 1I) under intraoperative image intensification and, if the distal incision can be
apposed easily without tension (Fig. 1J), direct primary closure can be performed. All incisions are reapproximated with a No. 2-0 nylon in vertical
mattress fashion and metallic skin staples with a suction drain placed in
the resultant dead space to limit the potential for hematoma formation
(Fig. 1K). The drain should be sutured at its distal end [56] and stapled at
the exit point from the skin to prevent it from being inadvertently removed
prematurely.

If the defect created following appropriate debridement precludes primary closure, filling the dead space with polymethylmethacrylate antibiotic-loaded bone cement beads is a useful technique and has been
described in depth in the literature [57–59]. The antibiotic beads usually
are removed and replaced during subsequent debridements in the operative
theater but can be left in place for 2 to 3 weeks if necessary. Intravenous -
antibiotics and any necessary local wound care are continued until the incisions are granular, at which point they can be covered with a split-thickness
skin graft that usually is harvested from the medial arch of the foot [60–63],
posterior calf [61–63], or thigh region of the ipsilateral limb [61,63]. The harvested split-thickness skin graft then is prepared for soft-tissue wound coverage by either fenestration of the graft manually with repeated passes of
a surgical scalpel (ie, pie crusting') or meshing it at a ratio of 1:1.5 or greater
using a commercially available mesher [63,64].

If it is not possible to primarily close the toe amputation incision, and the
ability to perform extended local wound care is inappropriate, the use of
mini-external fixation to assist in wound closure can be performed. This is
especially useful in patients who have noncompliant skin [4–7] or nonreconstructable peripheral vascular disease, where tension across the wound
would lead to necrosis [12,18,25].

Several techniques are possible, but the ones most commonly employed
involve mini-external fixation [46,47] or ring-type external fixation devices
[38,43,44]. With either technique, it is important to place a suction or gravity
drain in the dead space (Fig. 2A), and place all sutures for delayed closure of
the distal incision site (Fig. 2B). If the sutures are not placed at this time, it
will be exceedingly difficult if not impossible to reapproximate the skin edges
once the forefoot is narrowed sufficiently. For the mini-external fixation
device [46,47], one or two half-pins are inserted in the metatarsals adjacent
to the resected ray. It is important to insert these pins at the level of the surgical neck of the metatarsal (ie, metaphyseal–diaphyseal junction) to take
advantage of the distal lever arm, which allows more rapid approximation
of the metatarsals and therefore the intended soft tissues. The mini-external
fixation device then is compressed using the wrench as much as possible on
the operating room table but not so much as to fracture the metatarsals or
disrupt vascular flow. The mini-external fixation device then is compressed,
with advancement of the wrench every 24 to 48 hours until the skin edges are

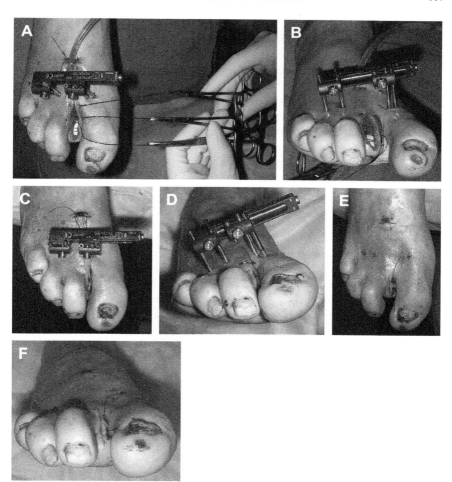

Fig. 2. Intraoperative anterior–posterior (*A*) and en fass (*B*) photographs demonstrating the use of a mini-external fixation device to facilitate close the distal incision through narrowing of the forefoot following minimum-incision ray resection. Note the use of a suction drain that has been stapled in place exiting through the dorsal incision to perform the metatarsal osteotomy and the placement of sutures through the distal incision, which will be used to formally reapproximate the skin edges after narrowing of the forefoot has been completed. Postoperative anterior–posterior (*C*) and en fass (*D*) photographs demonstrating closure of the distal incision and narrowing of the forefoot following-minimum incision ray resection. Postoperative anterior–posterior (*E*) and en fass (*F*) photographs following removal of the mini-external fixation device demonstrating complete healing of the distal incision and some sustained narrowing of the forefoot following minimum-incision ray resection.

fully reapproximated with no tension (Fig. 2C). At this time, the preplaced sutures are tied, with or without supplementation of metallic skin staples (Fig. 2D). The mini-external fixation device is left in place until the skin edges have healed fully, and the device is loosened gradually every 24 to

48 hours to make certain the reapproximated skin edges are able to mature and sustain tension. Once this occurs, the mini-external fixation device is removed in the clinic under aseptic technique (Fig. 2E, F) with the sutures and staples being removed sequentially over the next 2 to 3 weeks.

For ring-type external fixation, the foot is placed inside of a half-ring oriented 90° to the plantar aspect of the foot when viewed from a lateral direction and parallel with the intended direction of compression across the metatarsals when viewed from an anterior–posterior direction (Fig. 3A) [43,44]. Alternatively, a foot plate ring can be used, with the plantar aspect of the foot parallel to the long axis of the foot plate when viewed from a lateral view and the transosseous wires oriented parallel with the intended direction of compression across the metatarsals when viewed from an anterior–posterior direction [38]. If the foot plate ring is employed, the hindfoot must be incorporated and is stabilized with several crossed olive wires through standard pedal safe corridors about the calcaneus and talus. For either external fixation technique, one olive wire is placed from medial-to-lateral at the level of the distal metaphyseal–diaphyseal junction of the metatarsals, and another is placed from lateral-to-medial in this same region. Simultaneous tensioning of the forefoot wires allows for precise and gradual closure of the cleft foot deformity (Fig. 3B). However, on occasion, percutaneous osteotomy of the adjacent metatarsals is necessary to allow complete soft-tissue reapproximation, especially with large defects that have a higher incidence of wire pull-out and metatarsal fracture if the wires are

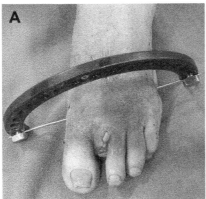 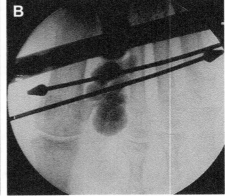

Fig. 3. Intraoperative photograph following application of a half ring oriented 90° to the plantar aspect of the foot and parallel with the intended direction of compression across the metatarsals (A). Note the complete apposition of the skin about the distal incision under no tension. Intraoperative image intensification view of the forefoot following minimum-incision ray resection demonstrating polymethylmethacrylate antibiotic-loaded bone cement beads within the second intermetatarsal space (B). Note the use of olive wires that have been cut flush with the olive bulb to allow placement under the skin edges and the location and orientation of the wires to facilitate forefoot narrowing.

overtensioned, especially in osteopenic bone. Because all interosseous compartments are passed through with either form of wire-based external fixation, compartment syndrome, nerve and vessel injury, and metatarsal fractures can be possible complications. The same sequence of events as described for postoperative treatment with use of the mini-external fixation device occurs with the ring-type external fixation devices described previously, although there is usually less of a need to slowly adjust the device.

With either external fixation technique, the patient is seen weekly for dressing changes and wire site care [64,65], which consists simply of cleansing the foot, ankle, and lower limb and external fixation device with antibacterial soap, followed by application of povidone–iodine solution to the pin–skin interface and a petroleum- impregnated gauze wrapped around each pin site followed by generous application of gauze pads fluffed and placed about the space created between the foot and external fixation device [66]. A bulky padded dressing [58] then is applied from toes to knee to limit edema, maintain hygiene, and limit the patient's direct view of the external fixation device, which improves tolerance during the fairly short recovery process while still permitting weigh sharing through a modified postoperative shoe application [45] if applicable. Once completely healed, appropriate postoperative shoe and orthoses or brace therapy is initiated and used by the patient along with proper pedal self-care and close follow-up on an indefinite basis [58].

Summary

Ulceration with infection and necrosis about the forefoot in high-risk patients represent significant challenges to the foot and ankle surgeon. The authors have presented a minimum-incision approach to metatarsal ray resection that allows minimum soft-tissue dissection, which preserves vascularity without compromising the intended goal of the procedure. This technique allows for precise narrowing of the forefoot without the need for osteotomy of adjacent metatarsals or their tarsal components and affords rapid healing by means of direct primary closure, application of a split-thickness skin graft, or use of mini- or ring-type external fixation to facilitate delayed primary closure. Minimum-incision ray resection is a safe, simple, reliable, and reproducible technique useful for treating localized toe and forefoot ulceration, infection, and necrosis that results in a stable, plantigrade, and functional foot.

References

[1] Frykberg RG. Diabetic foot ulcers: current concepts. J Foot Ankle Surg 1998;37(5):440–6.
[2] Isakov E, Budoragin N, Shenhav S, et al. Anatomic sites of foot lesions resulting in amputation among diabetics and nondiabetics. Am J Phys Med Rehabil 1995;74(2):130–3.
[3] Margolis DJ, Kantor J, Santanna J, et al. Risk factors for delayed healing of neuropathic diabetic foot ulcers: a pooled analysis. Arch Dermatol 2000;136(12):1531–5.

[4] Delbridge L, Perry P, Marr S, et al. Limited joint mobility in the diabetic foot: relationship to neuropathic ulceration. Diabet Med 1988;5(4):333–7.

[5] Mueller MJ, Diamond JE, Delitto A, et al. Insensitivity, limited joint mobility, and plantar ulcers in patients with diabetes mellitus. Phys Ther 1989;69(6):453–9.

[6] Fernando DJS, Masson EA, Veves A, et al. Relationship of limited joint mobility to abnormal foot pressures and diabetic foot ulceration. Diabetes Care 1991;14(1):8–11.

[7] Crisp AJ, Heathcote JG. Connective tissue abnormalities in diabetes mellitus. J R Coll Physicians Lond 1984;18(2):132–41.

[8] Armstrong DG, Stacpoole-Shea S, Nguyen H, et al. Lengthening of the Achilles tendon in diabetics who are at high risk for ulceration of the foot. J Bone Joint Surg Am 1999;81(4): 535–8.

[9] Armstrong DG, Stacpoole-Shea S, Nguyen H, et al. Lengthening of the Achilles tendon in diabetic patients. J Bone Joint Surg Am 2000;82(10):1510.

[10] Mueller MJ, Sinacore DR, Hastings MK, et al. Effect of Achilles tendon lengthening on neuropathic plantar ulcers: a randomized clinical trial. J Bone Joint Surg Am 2003;85(8): 1436–45.

[11] Ger R, Angus G, Scott P. Transmetatarsal amputation of the toe: an analytic study of ischemic complications. Clin Anat 1999;12(6):407–11.

[12] Nehler MR, Whitehall TA, Bowers SP, et al. Intermediate-term outcome of primary digit amputations in patients with diabetes mellitus who have forefoot sepsis requiring hospitalization and presumed adequate circulatory status. J Vasc Surg 1999;30(3): 509–17.

[13] Sommerlad BC, McGrouther DA. Resurfacing the sole: long-term follow-up and comparison of techniques. Br J Plast Surg 1978;31(2):107–16.

[14] Levin LS, Serafin D. Plantar skin coverage. Problems in Plastic and Reconstructive Surgery 1991;1(1):156–84.

[15] Levin LS. Foot and ankle soft-tissue deficiencies: who needs a flap? Am J Orthop 2006;35(1):11–19.

[16] Rosen RC. Digital amputations. Clin Podiatr Med Surg 2005;22(3):343–63.

[17] Bowker JH. Partial foot amputations and disarticulations. Foot Ankle Clin 1997;2(1): 153–70.

[18] Pinzur MS, Sage R, Schaegler P. Ray resection in the dysvascular foot. Clin Orthop 1984; 191:232–4.

[19] Pinzur MS, Sage R, Stuck R, et al. Amputations in the diabetic foot and ankle. Clin Orthop 1993;296:64–7.

[20] Smith DG. Principles of partial foot amputations in the diabetic. Foot Ankle Clin 1997;2(1): 171–86.

[21] Weinfeld SB, Schon LC. Amputations of the perimeters of the foot: resection of toes, metatarsals, rays, and calcaneus. Foot Ankle Clin N Am 1999;4(1):17–37.

[22] Quebedeaux TL, Lavery LA, Lavery DC. The development of foot deformities and ulcers after great toe amputation in diabetes. Diabetes Care 1996;19(2):165–7.

[23] Murdoch DP, Armstrong DG, Dacus JB, et al. The natural history of great toe amputations. J Foot Ankle Surg 1997;36(3):204–8.

[24] Benton GS, Kerstein MD. Cost-effectiveness of early digit amputation in the patient with diabetes. Surg Gynecol Obstet 1985;161(6):523–4.

[25] Shuttleworth RD. Amputation of gangrenous toes: effect of sepsis, blood supply, and debridement on healing rates. S Afr Med J 1983;63(25):973–5.

[26] Kerstein MD, Welter V, Gahtan V, et al. Toe amputation in the diabetic patient. Surg 1997; 122(3):546–7.

[27] Kaufman J, Breeding L, Rosenberg N. Anatomic location of acute diabetic foot infection: its influence on the outcome of treatment. Am Surg 1987;53(2):109–12.

[28] Armstrong DG, Lavery LA, Harkless LB, et al. Amputation and reamputation of the diabetic foot. J Am Podiatr Med Assoc 1997;87(6):255–9.

[29] Beyaert C, Henry S, Dautel G, et al. Effect on balance and gait secondary to removal of the second toe for digital reconstruction: 5-year follow-up. J Pediatr Orthop 2003;23(1):60–4.
[30] Little JM, Stephens MS, Zylstra PL. Amputation of the toes for vascular disease: fate of the affected leg. Lancet 1976;2(7999):1318–9.
[31] Greteman B, Dale S. Digital amputations in neuropathic patients. J Am Podiatr Med Assoc 1990;80(3):120–6.
[32] Seligman R, Trepal M, Giorgini J. Hallux valgus secondary to amputation of the second toe. J Amer Podiatr Med Assoc 1986;76(2):89–92.
[33] Pulla RJ, Kaminsky KM. Toe amputations and ray resections. Clin Podiatr Med Surg 1997; 14(4):691–739.
[34] Schweinberger MH, Roukis TS. Balancing of the transmetatarsal amputation with peroneus brevis to peroneus longus tendon transfer. J Foot Ankle Surg 2007;46(6):510–4.
[35] Schweinberger MH, Roukis TS. Intramedullary screw fixation for balancing of the dysvascular foot following transmetatarsal amputation. J Foot Ankle Surg 2008;47.
[36] Schweinberger MH, Roukis TS. Soft-tissue and osseous techniques to balance forefoot and midfoot amputations. Clin Podiatr Med Surg 2008;25(4):623–39.
[37] Köller A. Internal pedal amputations. Clin Podiatr Med Surg 2008;25(4):641–53.
[38] Zgonis T, Oznur A, Roukis TS. A novel technique for closing difficult diabetic cleft foot wounds with skin grafting and a ring-type external fixator. Operative Techniques in Orthopaedics 2006;16:38–43.
[39] Hansen ST Jr. Amputation techniques. In: Hurley R, Seigafuse SL, Marino-Vasquez D, editors. Functional reconstruction of the foot and ankle. Philadelphia: Lippincott Williams & Wilkins; 2000. p. 274–8.
[40] Anderson JJ, Woelffer KE, Holtzman JJ, et al. Bisphosphonates for the treatment of Charcot neuroarthropathy. J Foot Ankle Surg 2004;43(5):285–9.
[41] Strauss MB, Bryant BJ, Hart JD. Forefoot narrowing with external fixation for problem cleft wounds. Foot Ankle Int 2002;23(5):433–9.
[42] Armstrong DG, Wunderlich RP, Lavery LA. Reaching closure with skin stretching: applications in the diabetic foot. Clin Podiatr Med Surg 1998;15(1):109–16.
[43] Öznur A, Tokgözoğlu M. Closure of central defects of the forefoot with external fixation: a case report. J Foot Ankle Surg 2004;43(1):56–9.
[44] Öznur A. Management of large soft-tissue defects in a diabetic patient. Foot Ankle Int 2003; 24(1):79–82.
[45] Roukis TS, Zgonis T. Postoperative shoe modifications for weight bearing with the Ilizarov external fixation system. J Foot Ankle Surg 2004;43(6):433–5.
[46] Bernstein B, Guerin L. The use of mini-external fixation in central forefoot amputations. J Foot Ankle Surg 2005;44(4):307–10.
[47] Bibbo C. External fixator-assisted immediate wound closure. Techniques in Foot and Ankle Surgery 2006;5(3):144–9.
[48] Margolis DJ, Allen-Taylor L, Hoffstad O, et al. Diabetic neuropathic ulcers: predicting which ones will not heal. Am J Med 2003;115(8):627–31.
[49] Margolis DJ, Hoffstad O, Gelfand JM, et al. Surrogate end points for the treatment of diabetic neuropathic foot ulcers. Diabetes Care 2003;26(6):1696–700.
[50] Roukis TS, Stapleton J, Zgonis T. Addressing psychosocial aspects of care for patients with diabetes undergoing limb salvage surgery. Clin Podiatr Med Surg 2007;24(2):601–10.
[51] Öznur A, Özer H. Ray amputation with limited incision. Foot Ankle Int 2006;27(5):382.
[52] Roukis TS. Radical solutions: bold debridement techniques can work for both chronic and acute wounds. OrthoKinetic Review 2004;4(1):20–3.
[53] Levin LS. Debridement. Tech Orthop 1995;10(2):104–8.
[54] Attinger CE, Bulan E, Blume PA. Surgical debridement: the key to successful wound healing and reconstruction. Clin Podiatr Med Surg 2000;17(4):599–630.
[55] Attinger CE, Bulan EJ. Debridement: the key initial first step in wound healing. Foot Ankle Clin 2001;6(4):627–60.

[56] Dini GM, de Castilho HT, Ferreira LM. A simple technique to ensure drain fixation. Plast Reconstr Surg 2003;112(3):923–4.

[57] Roeder B, Van Gils CC, Maling S. Antibiotic beads in the treatment of diabetic pedal osteomyelitis. J Foot Ankle Surg 2000;39(2):124–30.

[58] Andersen CA, Roukis TS. The diabetic foot. Surg Clin North Am 2007;87(5):1149–77.

[59] Zgonis T, Stapleton JJ, Roukis TS. A stepwise approach to the surgical management of severe diabetic foot infections. The Foot and Ankle Specialist 2008;1(1):46–53.

[60] Roukis TS. Use of the medial arch as a donor site for split-thickness skin grafts. J Foot Ankle Surg 2003;42(5):312–4.

[61] Roukis TS, Zgonis T. Skin grafting techniques for soft-tissue coverage of diabetic foot and ankle wounds. J Wound Care 2005;14(4):173–6.

[62] Zgonis T, Stapleton J, Roukis TS. Advanced plastic surgery techniques for soft tissue coverage of the diabetic foot. Clin Podiatr Med Surg 2007;24(2):547–68.

[63] Roukis TS. Skin grafting techniques for open diabetic foot wounds and amputations. In: Zgonis T, editor. Surgical reconstruction of the diabetic lower extremity. Philadelphia: Lippincott Williams & Wilkins; 2008.

[64] Dahl AW, Toksvig-Larsen S, Lindstrand A. No difference between daily and weekly pin site care: a randomized study of 50 patients with external fixation. Acta Orthop Scand 2003; 74(6):704–8.

[65] Davies R, Holt N, Nayagan S. The care of pin sites with external fixation. J Bone Joint Surg Br 2005;87(5):716–9.

[66] Schade VL, Roukis TS. Use of a surgical preparation and sterile dressing change during office visit treatment of chronic foot and ankle wounds decreases the incidence of infection and treatment costs. The Foot and Ankle Specialist 2008;1(3):147–54.

ELSEVIER
SAUNDERS

Clin Podiatr Med Surg
25 (2008) 623–639

CLINICS IN
PODIATRIC
MEDICINE AND
SURGERY

Soft-Tissue and Osseous Techniques to Balance Forefoot and Midfoot Amputations

Monica H. Schweinberger, DPM, AACFAS, Thomas S. Roukis, DPM, FACFAS*

Limb Preservation Service, Vascular/Endovascular Surgery Service, Department of Surgery, Madigan Army Medical Center, 9040-A Fitzsimmons Avenue, MCHJ-SV, Tacoma, WA 98431, USA

Amputation is largely considered an undesired end point when treating limb-threatening conditions of the lower extremity. Although all reasonable attempts to preserve a patient's foot and lower leg should be considered, the functionality of the limb and likelihood of recurrent ulceration or infection must be assessed. In some cases, a well-balanced partial forefoot or midfoot amputation will provide the patient with a more durable extremity that will better maintain their independence than minimalistic procedures aimed at preserving a deformed forefoot.

Historically, forefoot and midfoot amputations were received negatively secondary to numerous complications that patient and surgeon encountered with them. Delayed or nonhealing of incision sites, re-ulceration, and recurrent infection are commonly reported following these procedures [1–3]. Poor long-term results of hallux amputations have been reported with re-amputation rates ranging from 53% to 61% in two retrospective studies [4,5]. Equinovarus deformity is a widely recognized complication of transmetatarsal and Lisfranc amputations often leading to recurrent ulceration and more proximal amputation [1,2]. Failure rates for transmetatarsal amputations (TMA) have been reported from 17% to 44% [1]. In looking critically at these complications, the majority of them can be traced back to three potential etiologies: (1) non-compliance; (2) multiple co-morbidities; and

Disclaimer: The opinions or assertions contained herein are the private view of the author and are not to be construed as official or reflecting the views of the Department of the Army or the Department of Defense.

* Corresponding author.

E-mail address: thomas.s.roukis@us.army.mil (T.S. Roukis).

0891-8422/08/$ - see front matter. Published by Elsevier Inc.
doi:10.1016/j.cpm.2008.05.006

(3) unaddressed pedal deformity [3]. Each of these is discussed in detail in this article.

Noncompliance

It is convenient at times to blame a patient's noncompliance with postoperative instructions for a poor outcome or undesired complication. Obviously, the patient must bear some responsibility if they willfully disregard their surgeons' orders despite warnings about the negative consequences, which include more proximal amputation. However, in many cases there may be barriers to compliance that should be identified preoperatively, or during the patient's hospitalization, and fully addressed [6]. The majority of patients undergoing amputation in the United States and Europe today are diabetic [7] and many are elderly, as well as, in poor physical condition. Postoperative, nonweight bearing restrictions may be impossible for these patient populations who therefore require alternative measures such as wheelchairs, total contact casts, or skilled nursing facility placement during recovery to protect the operative limb. If the patient lives alone at home, they may require a home health aide to help with their necessary activities of daily living, as well as, transportation to and from clinic appointments. Smoking cessation is imperative to improve the likelihood of incision healing [3] and patients may require referral to a smoking cessation support network to aid them in this process. Depression needs to be managed with counseling, support groups, or referral to a psychiatrist for evaluation and treatment, depending on the severity [3,6]. A social worker should be involved with every patient undergoing an amputation because failure to address the needs of the patient allowing them to maximize their ability to follow instructions will inevitably lead to postoperative complications.

Comorbidities

Medical comorbidities such as uncontrolled diabetes, peripheral arterial disease, chronic renal failure, and malnutrition all increase the risk of infection and nonhealing after partial foot amputation [3]. Uncontrolled diabetes impairs leukocyte function, which results in reduced host resistance and response to infection [8,9]. Peripheral arterial disease reduces the likelihood of incision healing secondary to inadequate perfusion of the surgical site [10]. Chronic renal failure causes proteinurea and resultant albumin deficiency, [3] which affects nutritional status and wound healing. Malnutrition can be precipitated by catabolism resulting from the presence of a wound or may pre-exist, before wound development. Regardless of the etiology, collagen synthesis is significantly impacted by inadequate nutrition [11].

In order to optimize the high-risk patient undergoing partial foot amputation and provide the most ideal conditions for successful postoperative healing without infection, multidisciplinary patient management involving endocrinology, infectious disease, internal medicine, nephrology, nutritional services, podiatric or orthopedic foot and ankle surgery, and vascular/endo-vascular surgery is required [12]. Significant patient education will likely be necessary to improve the patients overall health long-term.

Unaddressed deformity

Specifically in the neuropathic patient, ulcerations result from excessive, repeated pressure and shear on a concentrated area of the foot [13]. Defor-mities of the foot and ankle, such as equinus [14], hammer digit syndrome, hallux valgus, rigidly plantarflexed metatarsals, and Charcot neuro-osteoarthropathy deformity increase pressure and therefore the risk of ulcer-ation. Neuropathic patients with deformity and a history of ulceration have a 36 times greater risk for re-ulceration than the general population [15]. Hallux amputations have been demonstrated to cause increased pressure plantar to the metatarsal heads and toes compared with the contralateral side [16]. In addition, the severity of deformity on the contra-lateral limb worsens with time, especially at toes two and three and metatarsophalangeal joints two through five [17]. The increased plantar pressure and shear caused by this progressive deformity can result in both fracture and ulceration with potential infection and repeated amputation [18].

Equinovarus deformity seen after transmetatarsal and Lisfranc amputa-tions performed without proper balancing often results in ulceration at the plantar-lateral aspect of the stump from excessive pressure [19,20]. Follow-ing transmetatarsal or Lisfranc amputation, the foot is reduced in length leading to overpowering by the gastrocnemius-soleus complex, and the transverse arch of the foot is structurally aligned in varus due to the loss of the metatarsal heads. Therefore, the foot automatically assumes an equino-varus posture (Fig. 1). The equinus deformity will worsen if unad-dressed because of the elimination of extensor digitorum longus and exten-sor hallucis longus muscle function postoperatively, which causes an imbalance between the posterior compartment and the anterior compart-ment with resultant plantarflexion at the ankle joint [20]. Likewise, the varus deformity will worsen if left unaddressed secondary to the loss of intrinsic muscle function and disruption of the insertion of the plantar fascia causing subtalar joint imbalance and increased inversion pull of the tibialis anterior and posterior muscles, which overpower the eversion strength of the pero-neus brevis muscle [1]. Prophylactic surgery to correct deformity and reduce the likelihood of ulceration in neuropathic patients has been suggested by some authors [9,15].

When performing amputations, the surgeon must evaluate the patient's global foot structure and determine the etiology of the initial problem and what potential deformities may occur postoperatively. If each of the pa-tient's deformities and potential deforming forces is able to be surgically

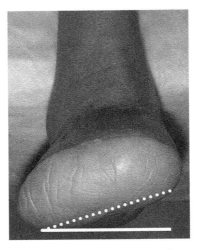

Fig. 1. Clinical en fass view following transmetatarsal amputation performed at another facility demonstrating the universal forefoot varus deformity present if soft-tissue or osseous balancing techniques are not employed.

addressed, the likelihood of recurrent ulceration and amputation should be reduced. This paper focuses on specific techniques to appropriately balance transmetatarsal and Lisfranc amputations with tendon transfer, as well as joint stabilization to consistently provide a stable, plantigrade, and functional residual foot.

Indications

The appropriate amputation level for an individual patient is determined by vascular supply, available soft tissue coverage, and deformity or previous surgery. An ankle brachial index (ABI) of ≤ 0.45 is generally considered incompatible with healing, while transcutaneous oxygen tension of ≥ 30-mm Hg or greater indicates, but does not guarantee, the potential to heal [3]. When a patient's arterial supply is in question, a vascular surgeon or endovascular specialist should be consulted to determine if revascularization procedures are indicated. The partial foot amputation must be performed at a level with adequate perfusion to heal.

Large open wounds on the dorsal or plantar foot must be excised before definitive closure of an amputation, and they may necessitate more proximal amputation if adequate soft-tissue is not available for coverage, especially plantarly. Primary closure is preferred; however, alternate methods of wound closure can be used if necessary. Skin grafts are generally thought to be a poor choice for coverage on weight bearing areas, but can be used in nonweight bearing areas of the plantar foot or dorsally for wound closure

[21]. Some surgeons will use skin grafting in weight bearing areas if there is adequate underlying granulation tissue and the patient can remain non-weight bearing on the foot until complete healing and maturation of the skin graft occurs at which point the tissue is quite durable. After they are fully matured, skin grafts usually contract a great deal, especially thin split-thickness skin grafts that can be excised and primary closed. Local flap coverage of plantar wounds may be possible depending on the size of the defect, mobility of the regional tissue, and adequacy of arterial supply to the foot [21,22]. Free flaps have been described, but can leave excessive bulk that is difficult to shoe or brace and prone to breakdown from the shear forces between the native and transferred tissue [23]. Performing the amputation at a level at which primary closure can be performed will avoid the additional incisions and potential vascular compromise associated with alternate wound coverage techniques and thus, may ultimately lead to a more functional and durable result.

In general, when a patient requires or has undergone a hallux or partial first ray amputation in isolation, owing to the high postoperative re-ulceration and re-amputation rates discussed earlier; has had two or more ray amputations; or has significant forefoot deformity in the presence of recurrent ulceration or infection, then a TMA or Lisfranc amputation should be considered. The amputation is performed at the most distal level compatible with healing and wound closure as discussed above [24]. Proper balancing of the residual stump will generally provide a durable, stable, plantigrade, and functional foot.

Forefoot and midfoot amputation balancing

TMA and Lisfranc amputations are routinely performed in conjunction with a percutaneous Achilles tendon lengthening, open gastrocnemius recession, or endoscopic gastrocnemius recession to address the equinus deformity. Details regarding procedure selection and techniques for soft-tissue ankle equinus correction can be found in a separate article included in this issue [25]. Additional tendon or osseous balancing is required to address or prevent varus deformity in both TMA and Lisfranc amputations. Some authors have recommended tenodesis of the flexor and extensor tendons from the 4th and 5th toes, while the foot is held in neutral position, to oppose the deforming forces of the gastrocnemius-soleus complex and tibialis anterior muscles [24]. This form of balancing is not recommended by the author as it leaves dysvascular tissue in the wound bed and does not have the strength or stability to balance the tibialis anterior or gastrocnemius-soleus complex. Split tibialis anterior tendon transfer (STATT) has been described to address forefoot varus after TMA and Lisfranc amputation [1]; however, this procedure requires three incisions and may be contraindicated in patients who have undergone peripheral arterial bypass surgery secondary to the potential for disrupting or compressing the bypass site which can lead to dorsal tissue necrosis. Peroneus brevis (PB) to peroneus longus (PL) tendon transfer can effectively plantarflex the first ray while simultaneously everting the forefoot after TMA, thereby, correcting the forefoot varus deformity [26]. However, this procedure may be contraindicated in patients with peripheral arterial disease due to the additional incision required and potential for wound dehiscence and delayed or nonhealing. An intramedullary screw placed through the residual first metatarsal or medial cuneiform and driven into the talus while the forefoot is held in neutral alignment, similar to the techniques described by various authors for percutaneous Charcot stabilization [27–31], can also correct forefoot varus and provide good stability to the medial column without the need for additional incisions [32]. This technique is effective for both TMA and Lisfranc amputations especially in patients with peripheral arterial disease [32]. Finally, transfer of the tibialis anterior tendon into the medial cuneiform and the peroneus brevis tendon into the cuboid [1,19] following Lisfranc amputation can maintain a rectus position of the foot post-operatively.

The three most commonly employed techniques by the senior author, (T.S. Roukis) are: (1) PB to PL tendon transfer, (2) intramedullary screw placement, and (3) transfer of the tibialis anterior tendon into the medial cuneiform and the peroneus brevis tendon into the cuboid. Each of these is discussed in detail in the following sections.

Peroneus brevis to peroneus longus tendon transfer

The surgical procedure begins with the patient positioned in the supine position on the operating room table with a well-padded bolster placed beneath the ipsilateral buttock to control physiologic external rotation of the lower limb. The incision is mapped out at the midpoint between the posterior edge of the distal tip of the lateral malleolus and the dorsal edge of the posterior aspect of the 5th metatarsal base and is approximately 3 cm in length (Fig. 2 A) [26]. A No. 10 blade is used to incise the skin approximately 1 cm in depth exposing the underlying peroneal retinaculum, which should be visible at the base of the incision. The peroneal retinaculum is then incised in line with the skin incision allowing visualization of the PL tendon inferiorly and the PB tendon superiorly. The intertendinous portion of the peroneal retinaculum is excised to facilitate the transfer. A clamp is placed about the PB tendon adjacent to its insertion on the 5th metatarsal base. The PB tendon is then transected distal to the clamp and retrieved from the surgical site. Electrocautery is used to mark the location of two longitudinal tenotomy incisions to be performed in the PL tendon through which the PB tendon will be weaved. Two stab incisions are performed with a No. 10 blade and then a 90° angled clamp is placed from deep to superficial to advance the PB tendon through the PL tendon at the proximal

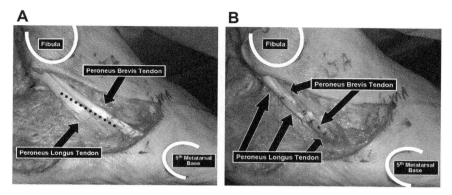

Fig. 2. (*A*) Photograph of a cadaveric specimen following resection of the soft-tissue about the hindfoot demonstrating proper skin incision placement (*black dotted line*) employed to access the peroneus brevis and peroneus longus tendons. (*B*) The peroneus brevis tendon has been weaved through the peroneus longus tendon and figure-of-eight locking sutures have been placed to maintain the transfer as discussed in the manuscript.

tenotomy site. A second 90° angled clamp is placed from superficial to deep through the distal tenotomy incision and used to grasp the PB tendon and advance it through this incision site. Distal tension is applied to the PB tendon with the residual forefoot held with the residual first metatarsal plantarflexed and the entire forefoot in eversion, thereby correcting the forefoot varus deformity. With the foot held in corrected position and distal tension placed on the transferred PB tendon, 2-0 Nylon suture is placed in a figure–of–eight locking pattern at the proximal and distal tenotomy sites incorporating both the PB and PL tendons in each area (Fig. 2 B). Once complete, a 3 cm x 3 cm piece of biologic tissue substitute (OrthADAPT Bioimplant; Pegasus Biologics, Inc., Irvine, CA) is wrapped around the conjoined PB and PL tendons and secured in place with 2-0 Nylon in a vertical mattress suture through only the biological tissue and some surrounding adipose tissue and not the transferred tendons. The use of biological tissue, as described, limits the potential for adherence of the tendons to the overlying skin, as well as functioning as a neosheath, which allows unimpeded gliding of the tendons. The surgical site is irrigated, a suction drain secured in place, and skin closure is performed with a combination of 2-0 Nylon in vertical mattress fashion and metallic skin staples [26].

Potential complications associated with this procedure include nonhealing of the incision site, tendon rupture, reaction to the implanted biomaterial, and infection. The procedure is contraindicated in the dysvascular foot due to a significantly increased risk of wound dehiscence. Postoperative care consists of nonweight bearing in a sugar-tong plaster splint or total contact cast for 4 to 6 weeks postoperatively, or longer, dependent on the rate of incision healing at both the tendon transfer site and the amputation stump.

A retrospective, observational cohort study was performed by the Limb Preservation Service at the Madigan Army Medical Center, Tacoma, Washington involving seven high-risk patients (nine feet) who underwent PB to PL tendon transfer as described above in conjunction with TMA (five feet) or reconstructive forefoot surgery (four feet). Three of the four feet undergoing reconstructive forefoot surgery had infected ulcerations on presentation. One female and six male neuropathic patients with a mean age of 66.1 years (range: 59 to 75 years) and a mean of 6.57 comorbidities (range: 4 to 12) were included. Eight of the nine feet healed the tendon transfer incision primarily. Complete healing with suture removal occurred in an average of 50.1 days [median: 47 days; range: 34 to 90 days]. The one patient who failed to heal primarily actively used tobacco products and repeatedly disregarded nonweight bearing instructions post operatively, returning for evaluation on multiple occasions with a wet, disheveled, and fractured total contact cast. All feet had adequate correction of forefoot varus deformity as evidenced by a plantigrade forefoot and lack of recurrent or de novo forefoot ulceration at a mean of 14.6 months postoperative (range: 10 to 18.5 months). One patient developed transient eversion weakness post operatively, which resolved with performance of physical therapy training at home.

Intramedullary screw fixation

Intramedullary screw fixation is indicated for balancing of the residual forefoot after TMA and Lisfranc amputation in patients with peripheral arterial disease who have a high-risk of wound dehiscence and in whom additional incisions should be avoided [32]. The procedure can be performed through the amputation incision site and therefore does not add additional wound healing risk to the patient. This technique must only be used when the surgical sites reveal no cardinal signs of infection or necrotic tissue.

The procedure is performed upon completion of the amputation and before wound closure. An assistant holds the foot in corrected position with the medial column plantarflexed and the forefoot in eversion to create a plantigrade residual foot. A guide wire for a large diameter cannulated screw is then placed through the medullary canal of the exposed 1st metatarsal or first cuneiform depending on whether a TMA or Lisfranc amputation was performed, respectively. The guide wire is driven across the articulations of the medial column into the talus with care taken to avoid inadvertent penetration of the ankle joint, especially medially (Fig. 3 A and B). The position is verified by intra-operative image intensification visualization of the foot and ankle (Fig. 3 C). Once the position is deemed appropriate, the bone is countersunk, the length of the screw is determined, and an appropriate length 8.0 mm cannulated titanium screw (Asnis III, Stryker Orthopaedics, Inc., Mahwah, NJ) is inserted until the head of the screw engages the subchondral bone of the first metatarsal, if present, or seated within the first

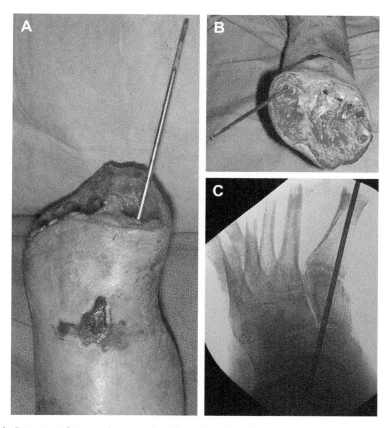

Fig. 3. Intraoperative anterior-posterior (*A*) and en fass (*B*) views following transmetatarsal amputation in a patient following below knee popliteal peripheral arterial bypass and percutaneous tendo-Achilles lengthening demonstrating insertion of a large diameter guide wire through the residual first metatarsal and into the talus. Note the gangrenous lesion overlying the dorsal midfoot that developed from pressure applied by a constrictive dressing over a 48-hour period. Intraoperative anterior-posterior image intensification view, confirming proper guide wire placement (*C*).

cuneiform in the case of a Lisfranc amputation. Drilling over the guide wire is not recommended before screw insertion as it will reduce screw purchase and stability. Allogenic bone graft (BioSet IC, RT Allograft Paste, Regeneration Technologies, Inc., Alachua, Florida) is placed over the implant and a biologic tissue substitute (OrthADAPT Bioimplant; Pegasus Biologics, Inc., Irvine, California) or the patient's abductor hallucis muscle is used to cover the end of the bone to protect the hardware from direct exposure in the case of wound dehiscence [32]. Alternatively, a 7.5 mm cannulated titanium threaded head screw (Charlotte Multi-Use Compression Screw System; Wright Medical Technology, Inc., Arlington, Tennessee) can be employed (Fig. 4), which has the added benefit of achieving

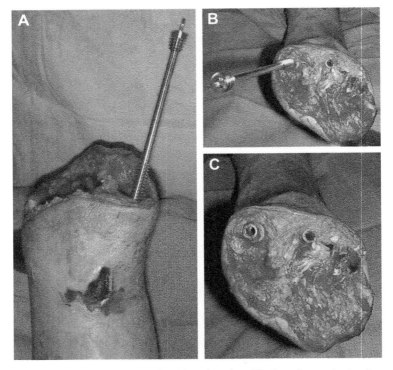

Fig. 4. Intra-operative anterior-posterior (A) and en fass (B) views demonstrating the proper length threaded head screw over the guide wire and fully seated within the residual first meta-tarsal (C).

compression across the medial column articulations without the need to fully seat the screw head and does not require the use of allogenic bone graft which reduces cost and complexity. Regardless of screw choice, the end result should be a stable and well-aligned forefoot (Fig. 5). Wound irrigation, suction drain placement, and skin closure is then performed as described above.

Potential complications of the procedure include infection, which could seed the retained hardware and spread along the cannulated portion of the screw into the hindfoot, as well as, iatrogenic fracture of the involved bones. Patients will have a stiff midfoot postoperatively, therefore, the hardware should only be placed after it has been verified that the foot is being held in fully corrected position. Nonweight bearing is required for 4 to 6 weeks postoperatively secondary to the adjunctive posterior lengthening performed, which is usually a percutaneous Achilles tendon lengthening (PTAL) rather than a gastrocnemius recession secondary to the patients poor vascular status [25] and to allow for incision healing at the amputation site.

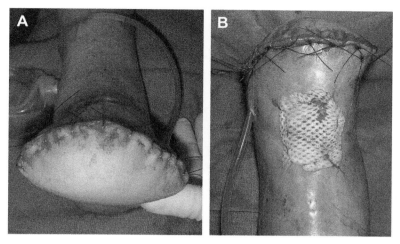

Fig. 5. Intraoperative en fass (*A*) and anterior-posterior (*B*) photographs following closure of the transmetatarsal amputation over a suction drain that has been sutured and stapled in place, as well as, débridement and coverage of the dorsal wound with a meshed cadaveric skin graft (GraftJacket Regenerative Tissue Matrix, Wright Medical Technology, Inc., Arlington, Tennessee). Note the rectus fore foot alignment achieved with the use of this technique.

Percutaneous extra-articular ankle immobilization can be performed in these patients to maintain the foot at 90° to the lower leg during healing of the PTAL procedure [33,34], because splint and cast application may be contraindicated after peripheral artery bypass surgery or due to prohibitive risk of ulcer development secondary to impaired arterial supply to the extremity. This procedure uses two smooth 2.8 mm Steinmann pins. The first pin is driven from the anterior-medial border of the distal tibia 5 cm proximal to the distal tip of the medial malleolus, posterior to the ankle and subtalar joints, and into the midportion of the posterior tuber of the calcaneus. The second pin is driven form the posterior-medial border of the distal tibia 5 cm proximal to the distal tip of the medial malleolus, anterior to the ankle joint, and ending in the neck of the talus or midsubstance of the navicular (Fig. 6) [34]. The pins are bent and capped or locked together with sterile self-adhesive dressing and then petrolatum-impregnated gauze is wrapped around the pin-skin interface followed by application of gauze between and around the pins. The patient must remain nonweight bearing on the extremity until pin removal at 4 to 6 weeks.

A retrospective case series was performed at Madigan Army Medical center involving five patients with diabetes and critical limb ischemia who underwent TMA for treatment of infected and or gangrenous toes with use of intramedullary screw fixation to correct forefoot varus deformity. Five males were included in this series with a mean age of 66.5 years (range: 59 to 75 years). The mean number of co-morbidities for this group was 6.5 (range: 4 to 8). All patients ultimately healed in a mean of 100 days (median: 85.5

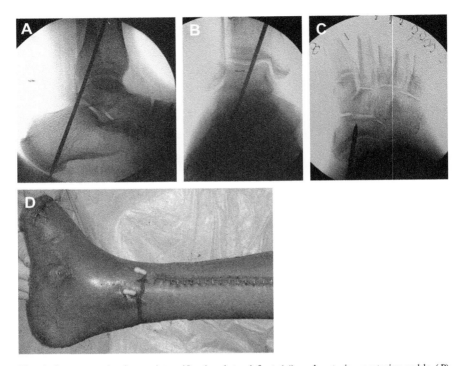

Fig. 6. Intraoperative image intensification lateral foot (A) and anterior-posterior ankle (B) views following insertion of the anterior-medial extra-articular pin, as well as, anterior-posterior foot (C) view following insertion of the posterior-medial pin in a patient who underwent a distal peripheral arterial bypass, percutaneous tendo-Achilles lengthening, and extra-articular pinning. Note the presence of a medial midfoot wound, which has been débrided and prepared for coverage with a meshed cadaveric skin graft (GraftJacket Regenerative Tissue Matrix, Wright Medical Technology, Inc., Arlington, Tennessee). Intraoperative medial view of the same patient following bending, cutting, and capping the extra-articular stabilization pins (D).

days; range: 52 to 180 days). Two of the five patients required a return to surgery for revision to a more proximal amputation secondary to ischemic complications of the residual forefoot. One had a re-stenosis of his posterior tibial artery and required repeat atherectomy before conversion to a Chopart amputation, as a result of ischemic compromise of the medial aspect of the plantar forefoot flap. Screw removal was necessary due to the proximal nature of the patient's final amputation level. It should be noted that the first dorsal metatarsal artery was transected during the original TMA and likely contributed to the patient's ischemic changes. Closure was obtained with application of a split-thickness skin graft over the distal stump. The second patient was converted to a Lisfranc amputation with maintenance of his medial column screw, which was simply advanced. Likewise, closure was obtained with application of a split-thickness skin graft over the distal stump. A third patient who was noncompliant with weight bearing restrictions, developed marginal

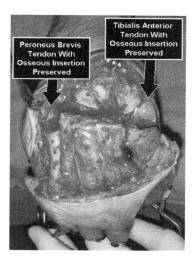

Fig. 7. Intraoperative en fass view of the foot following Lisfranc disarticulation with preservation of the tendinous insertion of the tibialis anterior and peroneus brevis tendons to the first and fifth metatarsal bases, respectively.

dehiscence of his incision and ultimately healed with local wound care while being treated at another facility. Each patient's foot demonstrated good correction of forefoot varus deformity upon postoperative evaluation and no hardware infections were encountered.

Anterior tibial and peroneus brevis tendon transfer

During amputations at the level of Lisfranc's joint, the insertions of the PB and tibialis anterior (TA) tendons are disrupted, which further weakens

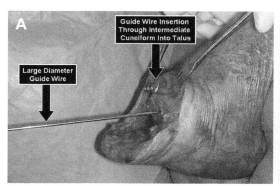
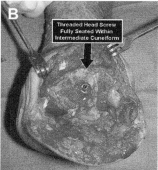

Fig. 8. Medial intraoperative view demonstrating proper placement of the guide wire through the intermediate cuneiform and into the talus (*A*) for a large diameter threaded head screw (Charlotte Multi-Use Compression Screw System; Wright Medical Technology, Inc., Arlington, Tennessee), which is recessed into the intermediate cuneiform (*B*).

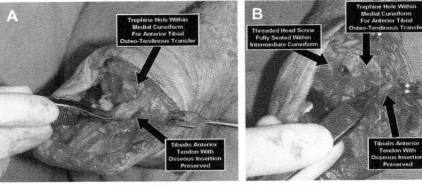

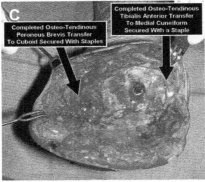

Fig. 9. Intraoperative views demonstrating distal traction on the anterior tibial osteo-tendinous transfer (*A*) followed by insertion into the trephine hole within the medial cuneiform (*B*). The same technique is employed for the osteo-tendinous peroneus brevis transfer into the cuboid. The osteo-tendinous transfers are then secured with one or more staples (Quick Staple, Wright Medical Technology, Inc., Arlington, Tennessee) to prevent pull-out (*C*).

the anterior compartment against the strong plantarflexory strength of the gastrocnemius-soleus complex. In addition, there is significant reduction in eversion strength because of the loss of PB muscle function with subsequent inversion of the residual stump by the unopposed force of the posterior tibial muscle. This reduction in strength can be prevented by PB and TA tendon transfer. Careful dissection is performed to disarticulate the tarsometatarsal joints while sparing the PB and TA tendon insertions. A sagittal saw can be used to osteotomize the base of the first and fifth metatarsals while preserving the attachment of the PB and TA tendons (Fig. 7). The remaining segments of the first and fifth metatarsals not attached to the tendons are removed from the surgical site along with the second, third, and fourth metatarsals. A large diameter screw is then inserted through the intermediate cuneiform and across the midfoot articulations into the talus using the technique described above to provide a stable midfoot (Fig. 8). With the foot held in corrected position and 90° to the lower leg, the PB and TA tendons are held taught and laid against the anterior aspect of the cuboid and medial cuneiform respectively to determine the appropriate location for attachment to provide adequate tension for tendon balancing. A trephine is then used to bore a hole into each of these areas and portions of the remaining bone from the first and fifth metatarsal bases are remodeled to fit into each respective bone tunnel. With the foot is held in corrected position the first metatarsal fragment, with TA tendon attached (ie, osteo-tendinous segment), is tamped into the medial cuneiform. The fifth metatarsal fragment with the PB tendon attached is then tamped into the cuboid [35]. One or two metal staples (Quick Staple, Wright Medical Technology, Inc., Arlington, Tennessee) are placed over the tendon transfer site and inserted to add additional tension and limit the potential for dislodgement of the transferred tendons (Fig. 9). Maintenance of the osseous insertion of these tendons allows bone-to-bone healing, which is more reliable and timely than tendon-to-bone healing, as well as technically more simple to perform. Wound irrigation, suction drain placement, and skin closure is then performed as described above (Fig. 10).

Complications associated with this procedure are fixation failure with loss of correction and delayed or nonunion of the transferred bone. Patients must remain nonweight bearing in a splint or cast, if indicated, postoperatively for 4 to 6 weeks or longer dependent on the rate of incision healing.

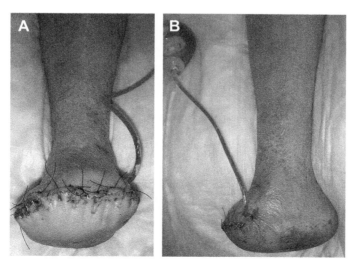

Fig. 10. Postoperative en fass (*A*) and medial (*B*) views following a well-balanced, rectus Lisfranc amputation using the soft-tissue and osseous techniques employed in the manuscript.

Summary

Performing a well-balanced transmetatarsal or Lisfranc's amputation as described here in a high-risk patient with multiple comorbidities can provide long-term mobility and independence. The lower energy expenditure required to ambulate with a partial foot amputation as opposed to a trans-tibial or trans-femoral amputation reduces cardiac stress, which may reduce mortality rates [1,36,37]. Avoiding multiple surgical procedures to amputate and re-amputate portions of the foot and the cumulative lengthy recovery time associated with this form of treatment, as well as the negative psychosocial impact to the patient, can also reduce perioperative morbidity. Proper surgical planning for the individual patient with involvement of social services and a multidisciplinary approach should provide the highest likelihood of success.

References

[1] Clark GD, Lui E, Cook KD. Tendon balancing in pedal amputations. Clin Podiatr Med Surg 2005;22(3):447–67.

[2] DeCotiis MA. Lisfranc and Chopart amputations. Clinc Podiatr Med Surg 2005;22(3): 385–93.

[3] Sullivan JP. Complications of pedal amputations. Clin Podiatr Med Surg 2005;22(3):469–84.

[4] Murdoch DP, Armstrong DG, Cacus JB, et al. The natural history of great toe amputations. J Foot Ankle Surg 1997;36(3):204–6.

[5] Greteman B, Dale S. Digital amputations in neuropathic feet. J Am Podiatr Med Assoc 1990; 80(3):120–6.

[6] Roukis TS, Stapleton JJ, Zgonis T. Addressing psychosocial aspects of care for patients with diabetes undergoing limb salvage surgery. Clin Podiatr Med Surg 2007;24(3):601–10.

[7] Armstrong DG, Lavery LA, Harkless LB, et al. Amputation and reamputation of the diabetic foot. J Am Podiatr Med Assoc 1997;87(6):255–9.

[8] Frykberg RG. An evidence-based approach to diabetic foot infections. Am J Surg 2003; 186(Suppl 1):44S–54S.

[9] Frykberg RG, Wittmayer B, Zgonis T. Surgical management of diabetic foot infections and osteomyelitis. Clin Podiatr Med Surg 2007;24(3):469–82.

[10] Hagino RT. Vascular assessment and reconstruction of the ischemic diabetic limb. Clin Podiatr Med Surg 2007;24(3):449–67.

[11] Arnold M, Barbul A. Nutrition and wound healing. Plast Reconstr Surg 2006;117(Suppl 7): S42–58.

[12] Andersen CS, Roukis TS. The diabetic foot. Surg Clin N Am 2007;87(5):1149–77.

[13] Bauman JH, Girling JP, Brand PW. Plantar pressures and trophic ulceration: an evaluation of footwear. J Bone Joint Surg Br 1963;45(4):652–73.

[14] Willrich A, Angirasa AK, Sage RA. Percutaneous tendo Achillis lengthening to promote healing of diabetic plantar foot ulceration. J Am Podiatr Med Assoc 2005;95(3):281–4.

[15] Simon SR, Tejwani SG, Wilson DL, et al. Arthrodesis as an alternative to non-operative management of Charcot arthropathy of the diabetic foot. J Bone Joint Surg Am 2000; 82(7):939–50.

[16] Lavery LA, Lavery DC, Quebedeax-Farnham TL. Increased foot pressures after great toe amputation in diabetes. Diabetes Care 1995;18(11):1460–2.

[17] Quebedeaux TL, Lavery LA, Lavery DC. The development of foot deformities and ulcers after great toe amputation in diabetes. Diabetes Care 1996;19(2):165–7.

[18] Rosenblum BI, Giurini JM, Chrzan JS, et al. Preventing loss of the great toe with the hallux interphalangeal joint arthroplasty. J Foot Ankle Surg 1994;33(6):557–60.

[19] Schoenhaus J, Jay RM, Schoenhaus H. Transfer of the peroneus brevis tendon after resection of the fifth metatarsal base. J Am Podiatr Med Assoc 2004;94(6):594–603.

[20] Reyzelman AM, Hadi S, Armstrong DG. Limb salvage with Chopart's amputation and tendon balancing. J Am Podiatr Med Assoc 1999;89(2):100–3.

[21] Levin LS. Foot and ankle soft-tissue deficiencies: who needs a flap? Am J Orthop 2006;35(1): 11–9.

[22] Zgonis T, Stapleton J, Roukis TS. Advanced plastic surgery techniques for soft-tissue coverage of the diabetic foot. Clin Podiatr Med Surg 2007;24(2):547–68.

[23] Hallock GG, Arangio GA. Free-flap salvage of soft tissue complications following the lateral approach to the calcaneus. Ann Plast Surg 2007;58(2):179–81.

[24] Attinger C, Venturi M, Kim K, et al. Maximizing the length and optimizing biomechanics in foot amputations by avoiding cookbook recipes for amputation. Semin Vasc Surg 2003; 16(1):44–66.

[25] Schweinberger MH, Roukis TS. Surgical correction of soft-tissue ankle equinus contracture. Clin Podiatr Med Surg 2008;25(4):571–85.

[26] Schweinberger MH, Roukis TS. Balancing of the transmetatarsal amputation with peroneus brevis to peroneus longus tendon transfer. J Foot Ankle Surg 2007;46(6):510–4.

[27] Grant WP, Sullivan RW. Medial column rodding for correction of the Charcot foot. In: Programs and abstracts of the American College of Foot and Ankle Surgeons 55th Annual Meeting and Scientific Seminar. Palm Springs: Fenruary 6, 1997. p. 13.

[28] Grant WP, Jerlin EA, Pietrzak WS, et al. The utilization of autologous growth factors for the facilitation of fusion in complex neuropathic fractures in the diabetic population. Clin Podiatr Med Surg 2005;22(4):561–84.

[29] Sammarco GJ, Guioa RG. Treatment of Charcot midfoot collapse with transverse midtarsal arthrodesis fixed with multiple long intramedullary screws Adelaide. Programs and abstracts of the Australian Orthopaedic Association. Referenced in J Bone Joint Surg Br 2004;86(Suppl 4):477.

[30] Zgonis T, Roukis TS, Lamm B. Charcot foot and ankle reconstruction: current thinking and surgical approaches. Clin Podiatr Med Surg 2007;24(2):505–17.

[31] Roukis TS. Minimally invasive soft-tissue and osseous stabilization (MISOS) technique for midfoot and hindfoot deformities. Clin Podiatr Med Surg 2008;25(4):655–80.

[32] Schweinberger MH, Roukis TS. Intramedullary screw fixation for balancing of the dysvascular foot following transmetatarsal amputation. J Foot Ankle Surg 2008.

[33] League A, Parks B, Öznur A, et al. Transarticular versus extra-articular ankle pin fixation: a biomechanical study. Foot Ankle Int 2008;29(1):62–5.

[34] Schweinberger MH, Roukis TS. Extra-articular immobilization for protection of percutaneous tendo-Achilles lengthening following transmetatarsal amputation and peripheral arterial bypass surgery. J Foot Ankle Surg 2008;47(2):169–71.

[35] Mommsen F. A new method of plastic tendon operation for the Lisfranc stump. Zentralbl Chir 1952;77(23):971–4.

[36] Pinzur MS, Gottschalk FA, Pinto MA, et al. Controversies in lower-extremity amputation. J Bone Joint Surg Am 2007;89(5):1118–27.

[37] Cutson TM, Bongiorni DR. Rehabilitation of the older lower limb amputee: a brief review. J Am Geriatr Soc 1996;44(11):1388–93.

ELSEVIER
SAUNDERS

Clin Podiatr Med Surg
25 (2008) 641–653

CLINICS IN
PODIATRIC
MEDICINE AND
SURGERY

Internal Pedal Amputations

Armin Koller, MD

*Department of Technical Orthopaedics, Münster University Hospital, Robert Koch Street 30,
48149 Münster, Northrhine-Westfalia, Germany*

"Amputation without amputation" or internal amputations are not a modern concept. Link in 1887 and Witzel and Hoffmann in 1889, when skeletal tuberculosis was a common problem, performed internal Chopart amputations. With the rarity of such conditions in the present day, internal Chopart amputation represents just one of myriad pedal amputation techniques that have fallen into oblivion [1]. Problems with the technically demanding fitting of prostheses or in-shoe orthoses resulted in a replacement of those procedures by standardized transtibial or transfemoral amputations. Vast improvements of prosthetics and custom shoemaking within the past few decades justify the reevaluation of individual and atypical resections and amputations possible within the foot.

A functional stump capable of accepting repeated weight-bearing is of utmost importance regarding lower extremity amputation surgery to afford the patient maximum mobility and self-dependence. The current thought process is to amputate as distal as possible to leave as long a foot segment as can safely be performed to enhance function, while employing robust tissues that have maximum healing potential to enhance durability. Additionally, the need to amputate and re-amputate should be avoided especially in patients with diabetes who have a higher mortality following major amputations, defined as above the ankle and more proximal, in comparison to nondiabetic amputees [2]. The existence of a lower limb amputation on one side is a statistical risk factor for a future contralateral amputation. In the presence of bilateral major amputation, loss of one knee joint most likely confines an elderly diabetic to the wheelchair [2]. Taken collectively, these are sound reasons to avoid amputations above the ankle joint if at all possible in the high-risk patient population.

Gangrene, as well as soft-tissue and osseous infections, are indications for partial foot amputations. Typically, stump coverage with plantar skin is

E-mail address: armin.koller@uni-muenster.de

doi:10.1016/j.cpm.2008.05.013

performed because this durable tissue allows for end-bearing capacity; however, to preserve maximum residual foot length, atypical coverage of the stump with dorsal skin is an acceptable alternative with good functional results [3,4].

The question arises: why sacrifice viable distal toes if the soft-tissue or osseous infection is limited to the tarsal or metatarsal bones? Osteomyelitis of the tarsal bones complicating a Charcot neuro-osteoarthropathy deformity is a condition that can be compared with the aforementioned bone tuberculosis. More than 100 years ago, surgeons performed intercalary bone resections of the tarsal bones (ie, internal pedal amputation), provided that the surrounding soft tissue was viable with success [1]. An internal pedal amputation represents a viable option for stable, durable, and functional limb salvage because most of the foreshortened feet following amputation can fit within custom-molded shoe-gear after the soft-tissue has stabilized. A distinction exists between three types of internal pedal amputations: 1) resection of all metatarsal and/or all tarsal bones (talus and calcaneus not included) with marked shrinkage of the foot; 2) intercalary resection of tarsal bones and arthrodesis with or without Kirschner wire fixation; and 3) resection of the talus with application of external fixation to achieve arthrodesis.

Internal transmetatarsal and tarsal-metatarsal amputations

The technique for an internal transmetatarsal amputation is performed through two parallel dorsal incisions. A soft-tissue bridge of ≥5-cm width is essential to limit the potential for skin necrosis between the incisions (Fig. 1). Using power instrumentation osteotomy is performed through each of the metatarsal bases to create a bevelled weight-bearing parabola. Following osteotomy, each of the metatarsals is freed from their soft-tissue attachments and removed from the surgical field. If necessary, the proximal phalanx to each toe can be resected, however, the remaining portions of the toes and all soft-tissue are preserved. Following full-thickness débridement of any open wounds to healthy bleeding tissue, the surgical sites are copiously irrigated with pulsitile lavage and a suction drain is placed along with polymethylmethacrylate antibiotic-loaded bone cement beads within the osseous void and left exiting the wound cavity [5]. The antibiotic bead chain is slowly removed over the next 10 to 14 days time. Resection and primary closure of any associated plantar wounds are not recommended because they tend to heal via secondary intent in concert with the impressive soft-tissue contracture that occurs over time (Fig. 2).

The technique for performing an internal tarsal-metatarsal (ie, Lisfranc) amputation involves the same surgical approach, employing two dorsal incisions, except that the lateral incision has is concave laterally for easier access to the base of the fifth metatarsal. The first, third, and fourth metatarsals are disarticulated at the tarsal-metatarsal joints. The second

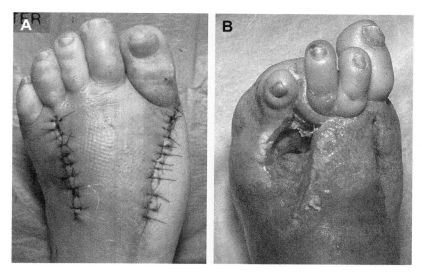

Fig. 1. (*A*) Parallel dorsal incisions for internal transmetatarsal and tarsal-metatarsal amputations maintaining a soft-tissue bridge of ≥5-cm width. (*B*) Skin necrosis due to insufficient distance between the incisions.

metatarsal, which resides with a deep recess between the medial and lateral cuneiforms, is osteotomized in line with the adjacent cuneiforms rather than disarticulated. If the cartilage is viable, as evidenced by a healthy white appearance and firm adherence to the bone, it is not resected because it serves as a natural barrier against contiguous spread of infection. The fifth

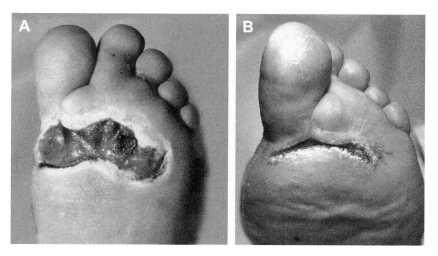

Fig. 2. (*A*) Large plantar ulceration and metatarsal osteomyelitis. (*B*) Soft-tissue contracture and ulcer healing via secondary intent.

metatarsal base is resected in subperiosteal fashion to preserve the attachment of the peroneus brevis tendon and limit the potential for a varus forefoot deformity (Fig. 3).

Internal midtarsal amputations

An internal midtarsal (ie, Chopart) amputation, the "Link-Witzel procedure," is associated with an extensive volume of bone loss, making meticulous drainage of the wound cavity is mandatory. This surgical procedure is performed on a patient-specific basis, so that a universal approach does not exist. Therefore incision location depends on the quality of the soft-tissue integument and the location of ulceration or gangrene. As with internal metatarsal or tarsal-metatarsal amputations, two parallel longitudinal incisions as advocated by Baumgartner and Greitemann [6] are preferred.

Postoperative treatment

A bulky, well-padded compressive bandage helps to avoid axial deviation of the forefoot during soft-tissue contracture of the residual forefoot. The

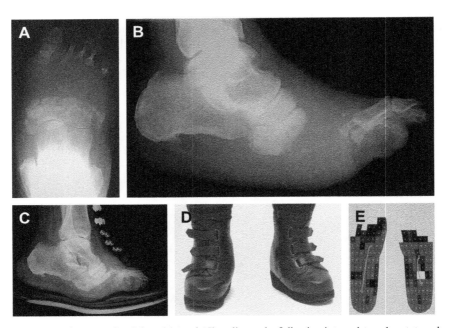

Fig. 3. Anterior-posterior (A) and lateral (B) radiographs following internal tarsal-metatarsal amputation. Lateral radiograph obtained within the shoe after significant soft-tissue contracture (C). Photograph (D) and plantar peak pressure distribution (E) with custom-molded multi-density shoe inserts following bilateral internal pedal amputation.

use of in-shoe orthoses is not necessary with internal transmetatarsal or tarsal-metatarsal amputation. Mobilization is begun in a postoperative shoe or custom-made interim shoe. In either case, the ongoing foreshortening of the foot necessitates frequent adjustments of the shoe. After several months, when the foot has achieved its final shape, a custom-molded shoe with stiff-rocker sole and reinforced heel counter which has proximally extended shaft above the ankle is fabricated because dorsiflexion and plantarflexion are not significantly restricted in this type of shoe. Following internal midtarsal amputation, a weight-bearing short-leg cast or ankle-foot orthosis is dispensed, and the patient is followed closely because modifications to the protective devices are frequently necessary. After full healing has occurred, a custom-molded high-shafted rocker bottom shoe with an extended, stiff tongue, is dispensed to further support the foot (Fig. 4).

Internal pedal amputations: intercalary resection

For an intercalary resection of tarsal bones, the author prefers a medial longitudinal incision for wide exposure. Following detachment of soft-tissue from the dorsal, medial, and plantar aspect of the foot in subperiosteal

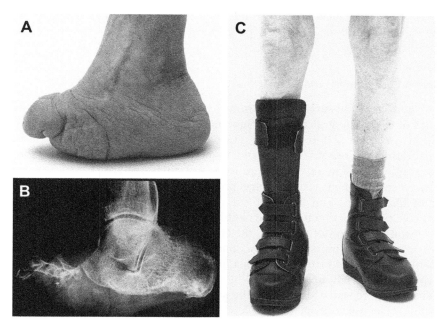

Fig. 4. (A) Lateral weight-bearing clinical photograph of a plantigrade foot following internal midtarsal (Chopart) amputation. (B) Lateral radiograph of the same patient demonstrating stable pseudo-arthrosis between toes and talus. High-shafted rocker bottom shoe with an extended, stiff tongue for the patient shown in Fig. 4 A and 4 B (C).

fashion, the infected bone is resected within two parallel osteotomies. Poly-methylmethacrylate antibiotic-loaded bone cement beads are packed within the osseous void for 14 days time to provide regional sterility after which they are removed during a second operation. During the second operation, two crossed Kirschner wires are placed extending from the forefoot into the rearfoot followed by application of a short-leg cast. The Kirschner wires are removed 6 to 8 weeks after the second operation and the patient immobilized in a short leg cast for an additional 6 weeks time or a custom device is fabricated consisting of either a Charcot-restraint orthotic walker (CROW) or a frame orthosis. With either type of custom device, weight-bearing is allowed 2 months postoperatively followed by transition into custom-molded shoe gear 5 to 6 months post operatively (Fig. 5).

With large ulcerative wounds, the author will first resect the ulceration and then resect the infected bone through the excised ulcer followed by pulsitile lavage with antibiotic solution and extensive débridement of the wound cavity. In this scenario, polymethylmethacrylate antibiotic-loaded bone cement beads are again packed within the osseous defect. On occasion, following removal of the antibiotic cement beads, the foot becomes quite stable during the contracture process such that further attempts at osteo-synthesis are unnecessary. The dead-space between the osseous ends within the foot narrows over time and frequently forms a stable pseudo-arthrosis. Following use of short leg cast for 3 months time, a postoperative shoe or custom-made interim shoe can be dispensed because the use of in-shoe orthoses is unnecessary (Fig. 6).

Internal pedal amputations: talectomy

Planning of the surgical incision depends on the location and character-istics of pre-existing ulcerations. Superficial ulcerations with healthy granu-lation tissue are left to heal via secondary intent whereas full-thickness, perforating ulcerations that extend to bone should be incorporated into the surgical incision and excised in toto. Although it is possible to perform these steps through a single-stage procedure, it is generally necessary to delay final closure and thus perform a series of staged procedures with the use of polymethylmethacrylate antibiotic loaded bone cement beads. Following resection of the talus, the ends of the medial and lateral malleoli are resected and morselized into bone graft unless they are infected. All cartilage is removed from distal tibia, navicular, and calcaneus, and the cor-tical bone is serially resected until bleeding cancellous bone is encountered followed by repeated drilling of the subchondral bone to further enhance healing. The tibia, navicular, and calcaneus are approximated with serial re-section occurring until all osseous components are in direct contact and the foot is plantigrade and aligned under the lower leg. The morselized bone graft is mixed with segments of a gentamicin-impregnated collagen sponge [7] and packed into any osseous defects. The critical component of this

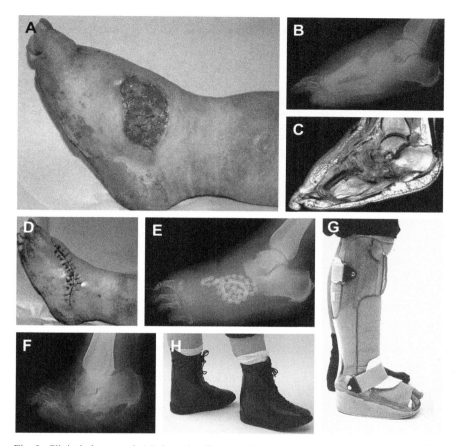

Fig. 5. Clinical photograph (*A*), lateral radiograph (*B*), and magnetic resonance imaging (*C*) of a massive soft-tissue infection with large ulceration and underlying osteomyelitis of tarsus and metatarsals. Clinical photograph (*D*) and lateral radiograph (*E*) following extensive osseous resection including excision and primary closure of the ulceration followed by insertion of polymethylmethacrylate (PMMA) antibiotic loaded bone cement beads within the osseous void. (*F*) Lateral radiograph demonstrating soft-tissue contracture one year after removal of the PMMA beads. (*G*) Postoperative mobilization by means of interim frame orthosis. (*H*) Final result in custom-molded multi-density shoe inserts with rocker soles.

procedure is proper foot alignment because osseous union between the tibia and calcaneus will occur with axial loading during use of the custom orthoses postoperatively [8]. Following osseous resection and alignment, an external fixator is applied consisting of a "box-shaped" design. Two, 250-mm centrally-threaded transfixion pins are drilled through the proximal tibia, one through the calcaneus, and one through the metatarsals followed by connection of the pins to the external fixation frame with four, longitudinal connection rods (Fig. 7).

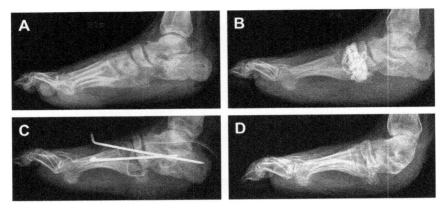

Fig. 6. Lateral radiograph demonstrating tarsal osteomyelitis (*A*), which was resected and packed with PMMA antibiotic-loaded beads packed within the osseous void after intercalary tarsal resection (*B*). Following removal of the PMMA beads the forefoot was docked to the rearfoot and stabilized with crossed Kirschner-wires (*C*). Lateral radiograph demonstrating solid osseous union and no signs of ongoing infection (*D*). Note that an additional partial calcanectomy had been performed due to calcaneal osteomyelitis and persistent heel ulcer.

Postoperative treatment

The external fixator is removed after 6 to 8 weeks, followed by use of compression therapy and short leg cast immobilization for 2 to 3 days to allow for fabrication of an interim ankle-foot orthosis. Axial compression within the orthosis allows for further compression between the tibia and calcaneus, which promotes osseous union or development of a stable

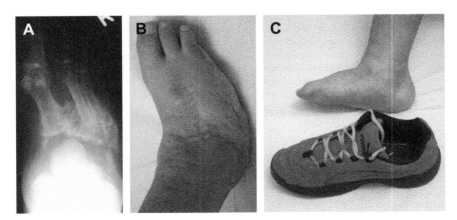

Fig. 7. Anterior-posterior radiograph (*A*) and clinical photograph (*B*) following intercalary tarsal resection and temporary placement of PMMA antibiotic-loaded beads. Plantigrade and stable foot without any ulceration 6 months after last operation despite wearing of commercially available sneakers without any inserts (against orders) (*C*).

pseudarthrosis (Fig. 8). Axial load transmission to the hindfoot is not only well tolerated, but is absolutely necessary to develop a sound connection between the foot and lower leg. The ankle-foot orthotic is continued for 9 to 12 months postoperatively after which custom-molded shoes are dispensed [8].

Discussion

Traditional "external" pedal amputations decrease the support surface area of the residual foot, which increases plantar pressure. This is amplified

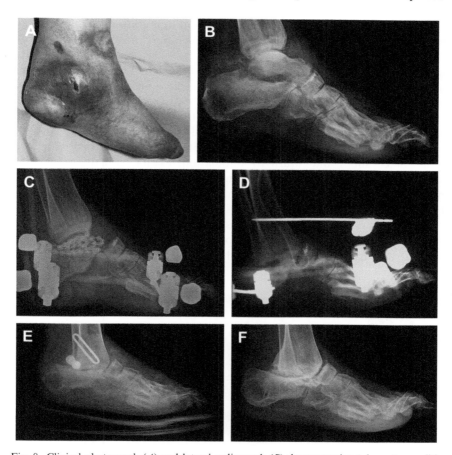

Fig. 8. Clinical photograph (*A*) and lateral radiograph (*B*) demonstrating talar osteomyelitis with discharging sinus. (*C*) Lateral radiograph following talectomy and partial resection of calcaneus and insertion of PMMA antibiotic-loaded beads and external fixation. (*D*) Lateral radiograph demonstrating tibio-calcaneo-navicular arthrodesis with autologous bone graft from medial and lateral malleolus. (*E*) Lateral radiograph demonstrating axial compression possible in frame orthosis, which enhances osseous union. (*F*) Stable pseudo-arthrosis allows for fitting of a custom-made orthopaedic shoe.

in the presence of an uncorrected deformity resulting from failure to appropriately balance the partial foot amputation. Under these [9–12] circumstances the partial foot amputation is exposed to maximum risk of ulceration and re-ulceration, as well as, potential for higher-level re-amputation [13]. In addition to preserving tibial length for energy-saving ambulation [14], the largest possible plantar support surface should be maintained. If the plantar skin is impaired, stump coverage with flaps from other regions of the foot is possible [15]; however, this usually requires use of thinner dorsal, medial, or lateral tissues, which are poorly suited for the force and shear associated with ambulation unless protected with an accurate fitting custom-molded shoe and in-shoe orthosis.

In contrast to the above, an internal pedal amputation has the advantage of simultaneously saving lever length, support area and plantar soft tissue. Drescher in 1990 and Baumgartner in 1994 reported good results following internal pedal amputations including complete removal of the metatarsal and tarsal bones [16]. A retrospective analysis of six patients with Charcot neuro-osteoarthropathy, who underwent an internal midtarsal amputation for chronic osteomyelitis of the tarsal bones and excision of associated plantar ulcerations and were followed for a mean of 55 weeks postoperatively, revealed that five of the patients could be fitted with custom-molded shoes and return to ambulation. Plantar soft-tissue scarring did not interfere with cosmesis or function, ulcerations and infection did not recur, and no further proximal amputation was necessary (see Fig. 8) [17].

Even after radical internal metatarsal and tarsal-metatarsal amputations active plantarflexion of the residual forefoot is possible to variable degrees (Fig. 9) and dynamic pressure distribution of the plantar surface of the

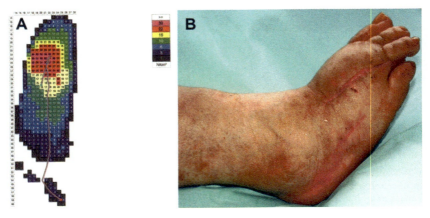

Fig. 9. (*A*) Barefoot plantar pressure distribution after internal midtarsal (Chopart) amputation. Note that the toes are to the bottom in Fig. 9 A. (*B*) Corresponding clinical picture demonstrates a stable, durable, and functional foot.

foot measured on a platform (E-med, Novel, Münich, Germany) occasionally reveals a gait pattern and pressure distribution resembling an intact foot. Within a year, the residual forefoot will contract such that the toes contact the remaining midfoot and become quite stable resembling a stable pseudarthrosis. A similar result frequently occurs with internal midtarsal amputations regardless of whether Kirschner-wire fixation was employed. This flexibility in the midtarsal area is considered advantageous since it allows for a smooth, even "roll-off," which reduces plantar pressure at the forefoot and bending moments at proximal pedal joints often seen with a long-stiff foot.

The psychologic impact of partial foot amputation is multifaceted and either transient or permanent depressive disorders occur in 23%–35% undergoing lower limb amputation [18]. However, following internal pedal amputations, patients do not believe that they have undergone a formal amputation and that stigmatization by the shortened foot was sensed less serious than if they did not have their residual toes [17]. Furthermore, the use of custom-molded shoes and in-shoe orthoses is well accepted by the patients following internal pedal amputation.

Soft-tissue imbalance is a common problem following partial foot amputation that requires a detailed evaluation and surgical management [9–12]. Internal pedal amputations frequently require transection of soft-tissue tendinous structures that cannot be re-attached or transferred, however, because the forefoot is mostly soft-tissue and the resected tendons are less likely to fully retract, a fairly well-balanced residual foot usually remains. Despite the shortened lever-arm that reduces the dorsiflexion force about the forefoot, soft-tissue equinus contraction does not occur as a consequence of internal pedal amputations that universally retain a plantigrade position [17]. Following internal pedal amputations, formal attempts at arthrodesis of the distal and proximal segments could be attempted with the use of internal compression or external fixation; however, it does not appear that this is necessary because a stable pseudarthrosis is more than sufficient to provide a stable, durable, and functional foot. Furthermore, the use of internal compression fixation permanently compromises the regional bone, which can be problematic in the face of previous infection because it blunts the natural ability to resist and treat infection, and bacterial biofilm may develop on metal surfaces and lead to a chronic and destructive infection [19]. Impairment of periosteal blood supply following implantation of metallic fixation may interfere with humoral and immunologic host defense mechanisms against the spread and multiplication of persistent microorganisms at the bone-implant interface [20]. In contrast to Kirschner wire transfixion, the use of an external fixation device allows for stability while avoiding metallic fixation within or across the internal amputation sites, which limits the potential for contiguous spread throughout the remaining foot skeleton. A minor disadvantage of external fixation is the rather laborious postoperative treatment care plan and difficulty associated with revision of the internal pedal amputation if infection progresses. According to literature, external fixation surgery for arthrodeses of the diabetic neuropathic ankle joint is marked with the blemish of increased infection rate [21,22]. A retrospective study on 65 Charcot feet operated in the authors' clinic did not support this statement because the presence of osteitis preoperatively did not negatively affect final outcome [23].

Summary

Internal pedal amputations, although not commonly performed, represent an elegant approach to severe soft-tissue and osseous infections throughout the foot skeleton capable of eradicating infection and producing a stable, plantigrade residual foot that can be properly placed into custom-molded shoe gear with either external or in-shoe orthoses. Formal arthrodesis across the resected segments is not necessary for a favorable outcome, as the development of a stable pseudarthrosis offers an adequate degree of stability. The ability to achieve these results without the need for permanent internal fixation is beneficial because future problems such as perforating ulcerations or osteomyelitis are less disastrous and easier to manage. The use of internal pedal amputations, as well as a structured postoperative treatment plan, allow for maximum functional limb preservation and associated improved patient outcomes.

References

[1] Petersen H, Gocht H. Amputationen und Exartikulationen. In: Bruns P, editor. Deutsche Chirurgie. Stuttgart (Germany): Enke; 1907.

[2] Schofield CJ, Libby G, Brennan GM, et al. Mortality and hospitalization in patients after amputation: a comparison between patients with and without diabetes. Diabetes Care 2006;29(10):2252–6.

[3] Harris RI. Symés amputation: the technical details essential for success. J Bone Joint Surg Br 1956;38(3):614–32.

[4] Koller A, Hafkemeyer U, Wetz HH. Syme amputation in heel defects. Orthopade 2001; 30(3):145–9.

[5] Evans RP, Nelson CL. Gentamicin-impregnated polymethylmethacrylate beads compared with systemic antibiotic therapy in the treatment of chronic osteomyelitis. Clin Orthop Relat Res 1993;295:37–42.

[6] Baumgartner R, Greitemann B. Die Resektion von Mittelfußknochen als Alternative zur Vorfußamputation. Oper Orthop Traumatol 1994;6:119–31.

[7] Mendel V, Simanowski HJ, Scholz HC, et al. Therapy with gentamicin-PMMA beads, gentamicin-collagen sponge, and cefazolin for experimental osteomyelitis due to Staphylococcus aureus in rats. Arch Orthop Trauma Surg 2005;125(6):363–8.

[8] Koller A, Meissner S, Podella M, et al. Orthotic management of Charcot feet after external fixation surgery. Clin Podiatr Med Surg 2007;24(3):583–99.

[9] Schweinberger MH, Roukis TS. Balancing of the transmetatarsal amputation with peroneus brevis to peroneus longus tendon transfer. J Foot Ankle Surg 2007;46(6):510–4.

[10] Schweinberger MH, Roukis TS. Intramedullary screw fixation for balancing of the dysvascular foot following transmetatarsal amputation. J Foot Ankle Surg 2008.

[11] Schweinberger MH, Roukis TS. Surgical correction of soft-tissue ankle equinus contracture. Clin Podiatr Med Surg 2008;25(4):571–85.

[12] Schweinberger MH, Roukis TS. Soft-tissue and osseous techniques to balance forefoot and midfoot amputations. Clin Podiatr Med Surg 2008;25(4):623–39.

[13] Armstrong DG, Lavery LA. Plantar pressures are higher in diabetic patients following partial foot amputation. Ostomy Wound Manage 1998;44(3):30–6.

[14] Wagner FW. Amputationen am Fuß bei Gefäßpatienten. Medizinisch-Orthopädische Technik 1984;1:10–3 [in German].

[15] Chang BB, Bock DE, Jacobs RL, et al. Increased limb salvage by the use of unconventional amputations. J Vasc Surg 1994;19(2):341–9.

[16] Drescher H, Wetz HH, Baumgartner R. Die Mittelfußknochenresektion zur Therapie des Malum perforans. Medizinisch-Orthopädische Technik 1990;110:12–9 [in German].

[17] Koller A, Wetz HH. Link-Witzel operation for diabetics. Orthopade 2003;32(3):231–5.

[18] Lange C, Heuft G. Coping with illness and psychotherapy for patients after amputation. Orthopade 2001;30(3):155–60.

[19] Costerton JW. Biofilm theory can guide the treatment of device-related orthopaedic infections. Clin Orthop Relat Res 2005;437:7–11.

[20] Arens S, Kraft C, Schlegel U, et al. Susceptibility to local infection in biological internal fixation: experimental study of open versus minimally invasive plate osteosynthesis in rabbits. Arch Orthop Trauma Surg 1999;119(1):82–5.

[21] Weber M, Schwer H, Zilkens KW, et al. Tibio-calcaneo-naviculo-cuboidale arthrodesis: 6 patients followed for 1-8 years. Acta Orthop Scand 2002;73(1):98–103.

[22] Stuart MJ, Morray BE. Arthrodeses of the diabetic neuropathic ankle joint. Clin Orthop 1990;253:209–11.

[23] Koller A, Hafkemeyer U, Fiedler R, et al. Reconstructive foot surgery in cases of diabetic-neuropathic osteoarthropathy. Orthopade 2004;33(9):983–91.

ELSEVIER
SAUNDERS

Clin Podiatr Med Surg
25 (2008) 655–680

CLINICS IN
PODIATRIC
MEDICINE AND
SURGERY

Minimally Invasive Soft-Tissue and Osseous Stabilization (MISOS) Technique for Midfoot and Hindfoot Deformities

Thomas S. Roukis, DPM, FACFAS

*Limb Preservation Service, Vascular/Endovascular Surgery Service, Department of Surgery,
Madigan Army Medical Center, 9040-A Fitzsimmons Avenue,
MCHJ-SV, Tacoma, WA 98431, USA*

Unstable deformities in the midfoot and hindfoot represent significant challenges for the foot and ankle surgeon. The goal for any treatment regime involving these deformities is to create a plantigrade, stable, and shoeable/braceable foot, free from significant risk for further breakdown, recurrence, ulceration, and/or infection [1–12]. The choice between conservative and surgical intervention depends on the assessment of the risks and benefits of each. The "lesser of two evils" is usually applicable when one has to choose between conservative care using immobilization with strict nonweight bearing (ie, reliance on casting or bracing to maintain reduction, skin breakdown, deep venous thrombosis) and surgical intervention (ie, incision breakdown, infection, hardware failure) [13]. Unstable midfoot and hindfoot deformities are exceedingly difficult to correct surgically because of the relatively inflexible soft tissues about the midfoot and hindfoot, especially laterally, which make primary closure without tension at the time of surgical intervention difficult and the incidence of dehiscence high [13–16]. Primary healing of these deformities is also made more difficult by other factors for delayed wound healing associated with the high-risk patient such as poorly controlled diabetes, immunosuppression, corticosteroid use, renal disease, peripheral vascular disease, venous or lymphatic disease/edema, cardiac disease, malnutrition, noncompliance, psychosocial

---

The opinions or assertions contained herein are the private view of the author and are not to be construed as official or reflecting the views of the Department of the Army or the Department of Defense.

E-mail address: thomas.s.roukis@us.army.mil

0891-8422/08/$ - see front matter. Published by Elsevier Inc.
doi:10.1016/j.cpm.2008.05.005

issues [17–20]. Regardless of what conservative or surgical approach is employed, the worst case scenario must be assumed and the treatment plan made as "patient-proof" as possible.

The author presents a review of surgical approaches to the midfoot and hindfoot deformities with a focus on the high-risk patient, as well as the author's proposed surgical intervention through the use of a minimally invasive soft-tissue and osseous stabilization approach (MISOS), related in a detailed step-by-step fashion.

Historical review

The mainstay of surgical approaches to the midfoot and hindfoot involve a series of rather lengthy surgical incisions about the medial, dorsal-medial, dorsal, dorsal-lateral, or lateral aspects of the foot depending on the osseous structures surgery is intended to address [8,14,15,21]. The vascular supply to the foot has been evaluated in detail (Fig. 1A) and the "safest" incision placement has been inferred based upon the angiosome concept [22–25]. The term "angiosome" is defined as the composite block of tissue that

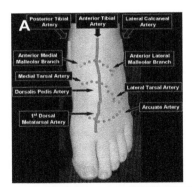

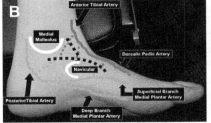 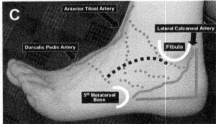

Fig. 1. (A) Anterior-posterior photograph demonstrating the vascular anatomy of the left foot and ankle with the interconnections between the main arterial segments (dotted lines). (B) Medial view of the left foot and ankle demonstrating the surgical incisions described to access the medial aspect of the midfoot and hindfoot (black hashed line). (C) Lateral view of the left foot and ankle demonstrating the purported safest surgical incision to access the subtalar and calcaneal-cuboid joints including the sinus tarsi (black hashed line) and calcaneus (solid gray line).

a dominant perforating vessel, which arises from an underlying source artery, supplies [26]. For the medial aspect of the midfoot and hindfoot, the purported safest surgical incision is placed 2 to 3 cm dorsal to the glabrous junction between the skin at the dorsal and plantar aspect of the foot that lies between the superficial branch of the medial plantar artery and the dorsalis pedis artery angiosomes (Fig. 1B) [24,25]. For the lateral aspect of the midfoot and hindfoot, two incisions are possible based upon the whether access is required to the calcaneus or the subtalar and calcaneal-cuboid joints including the sinus tarsi (Fig. 1C) [24,25]. The purported safest surgical incision to access the calcaneus is placed along the glabrous junction between the skin at the dorsal and plantar aspect of the foot that lies between the dorsalis pedis artery and lateral plantar artery angiosomes (see Fig. 1C). The purported safest surgical incision to access the subtalar and calcaneal-cuboid joints including the sinus tarsi is a horizontal incision placed directly over the sinus tarsi, which lies between the anterior tibial artery/dorsalis pedis and the perforating branch of the peroneal artery and the lateral calcaneal artery (see Fig. 1C). The incision can be extended distally to expose the calcaneal-cuboid joint if care is taken not to disrupt the lateral tarsal and arcuate arteries [24,25].

When visualizing these incisions, it is clear that they coincide with the traditional surgical approaches used [8,14,15,21], however, the purported safest surgical incisions are shorter and the soft-tissue dissection technique recommended more direct [24,25]. One must recognize that extending the incisions to coincide with the traditional surgical approaches violates the anastomoses between the angiosomes, which can lead to wound healing related issues secondary to tissue ischemia [24,25]. In addition to disruption of the cutaneous vascular supply about the surgical incisions, the vascular supply to the underlying osseous structures are also disrupted making osseous healing difficult to achieve in a timely fashion if at all. This is supported in the literature where it is generally accepted that midfoot and hindfoot arthrodesis are fraught with complications including risk of nonunion, infection, and avascular necrosis to name but a few [16,27–30]. The overall complication rate for midfoot and hindfoot arthrodesis procedures has been reported to be between 16% and 30% [27–32]. It should be noted that these studies involve a generally healthy patient population and not the high-risk patient that is at much greater risk of soft-tissue healing relates issues and osseous failure associated with delayed union, nonunion, and pseudarthrosis [33].

Recently, the use of an isolated extensile medial incision to perform arthrodesis of the midfoot and hindfoot articulations has been presented including some limited patient follow-up data [14,15]. Of note, none of the patients developed a wound-related problem about the medial aspect of the foot and the surgical re-alignment was deemed comparable to that achieved with the traditional dual medial and lateral incision approach. However, the intraoperative photographs depict an incision much longer than the one advocated above, as well as extensive manipulation of the soft-tissues to adequately expose the underlying osseous structures for the intended surgical correction. This approach is useful when treating severe, chronic, rigid dorsal-lateral peritalar subluxation (ie, pes plano valgus) deformities where use of a lateral skin incision has a high-risk of failure. The additional use of external fixation to provide osseous compression, assist with intraoperative re-alignment, and facilitate mobilization should be considered when applicable (Fig. 2).

Minimally invasive soft-tissue and osseous stabilization

The term "minimally invasive soft-tissue and osseous stabilization" defines a constellation of soft-tissue and osseous techniques employed to

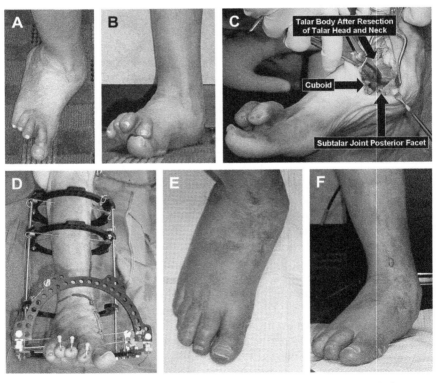

Fig. 2. Anterior-posterior (A) and en fass (B) views of the right foot demonstrating a severe, rigid, chronic, dosal-lateral peritalar subluxation deformity in an immunocompromised patient with a connective tissue disorder. Intraoperative photograph of the isolated extensile medial incision used to perform a triple arthrodesis facilitated by resection of the talar head and a portion of the neck (C), which facilitated reduction and alignment with a ring-type external fixation device, which permitted early mobilization (D). Postoperative anterior-posterior (E) and en fass (F) photographs demonstrating adequate realignment sufficient to use over-the-counter shoe gear with accommodative in-shoe orthoses.

create a well-aligned, stable, plantigrade, and functional foot and ankle capable of being placed into custom shoe gear with an accommodative in-shoe orthoses or brace. The main theme consists of minimal incisions with limited soft-tissue dissection through the use of topographic anatomic landmarks and image intensification, as well as the use of remotely delivered and stout internal fixation supplemented with biologic technology to enhance primary healing. A sound working knowledge of traditional open approaches to midfoot and hindfoot deformities is a prerequisite to attempting MISOS techniques. The MISOS approach should be reserved for the high-risk patient who would be unable to successfully heal traditional time-honored soft-tissue approaches and osseous preparation techniques.

With the patient positioned on the operating room table in the supine position and a well-padded gel bolster placed under the ipsilateral buttock to control physiologic external rotation of the lower limb the foot, ankle, lower leg, and thigh is prepped and draped in aseptic technique. A tourniquet is not necessary due to the limited soft-tissue dissection using well-placed incisions that respect the regional vascular structures. The author has found it useful to have the contralateral limb placed on an extra arm-board secured to the end of the table to provide additional working space for necessary instruments that can be placed between the limbs, as well as, allows clearance for placement of the intraoperative image intensification that is necessary throughout the procedure.

Unstable midfoot and hindfoot deformities are invariably associated with concomitant soft-tissue and osseous deformities of the lower leg (ie, ankle equinus contracture), forefoot (ie, sagital and/or transverse plane structural metatarsal deformities), and digital contractures [8,13]. The author's approach is to initially address the most proximal deformity and then progress distally until the entire foot, ankle, and lower leg is structurally aligned and functionally competent.

First, the equinus contracture that is nearly universally present [13,34] is addressed through either a percutaneous tendo-Achilles triple hemi-section, open or endoscopic gastrocnemius recession (A.M. Surgical Endoscopic Release System, Wright Medical Technology, Inc., Arlington, Tennessee) [35–37]. The endoscopic approach is the author's preferred method in nonspastic deformities with adequate perfusion because the correction obtained is comparable to a tendo-Achilles lengthening, but the potential for over-lengthening, rupture, and neurologic injury to the sural nerve is markedly reduced [37]. The only concern with the endoscopic gastrocnemius recession is the need to use a tourniquet to allow sufficient visualization. The indications, contra-indications, and specific techniques along with the "pearls for success" advocated and used by the author are published in this issue and will not be repeated here [37]. The goals of these procedures are to restore dorsiflexion of the foot at the ankle to 90° realizing that some additional correction occurs throughout the early postoperative period as the patient flexes and extends their knee which creates tension on the gastrocnemius and therefore the aponeurosis and Achilles tendon, as well as when they begin to ambulate. By resolving the equinus contracture, even the most contracted midfoot and hindfoot deformities will develop some laxity allowing partial reduction through application of the manual reduction techniques described below.

The posterior tibial tendon is then evaluated to determine if any contracture is present that can be contributing to the deformity and, if identified, it is released through a minimum incision based upon regional topography [38]. The posterior tibial tendon is easily identified by first marking out the medial malleolus and the navicular tuberosity and then palpating the space between the most anterior-distal aspect of the medial malleolus and the posterior-superior aspect of the navicular tuberosity. The bulk of the posterior tibial tendon courses directly between an imaginary line connecting these easily identified locations. A small linear incision is made through the skin at the center of the imaginary line until the posterior tibial tendon sheath has been identified. The sheath is initially incised in line with the skin incision and protected for later re-approximation after which the posterior tibial tendon is retrieved through the incision and sharply transected. The foot is then manipulated into eversion and dorsiflexion to release any adhesions between the posterior tibial tendon and the sheath and correction assessed. If the foot cannot be corrected to neutral alignment the talar-navicular joint capsule and components of the spring ligament can be transected under image intensification with a No. 64 Beaver blade or sharp narrow osteotome. At this point, it should be possible to fully reduce the foot to neutral alignment, which will be stabilized using the minimally invasive osseous stabilization technique described below. Following release of the posterior tibial tendon with or without talar-navicular joint capsulotomy and spring ligament release, the skin edges are re-approximated with a single vertical mattress suture of No. 2-0 Nylon incorporating the posterior tibial tendon sheath into the suture to limit the potential for formation of a tenosynovial fluid leak induced dehiscence or fistula. Dehiscence or formation of a fistula associated with tenosynovium is notoriously difficult to treat and frequently requires multiple attempts at revision to remove the sheath and productive tenosynovium. It is best to avoid this complication through the use of anatomic dissection and secure closure.

The peroneal tendons are then evaluated to determine if any contracture is present that can be contributing to the deformity and if identified, the tendons are released through a minimum incision based upon regional topography. The peroneal tendons are easily identified by first marking out the lateral malleolus and the 5th metatarsal styloid process and then palpating the space between the most posterior-distal aspect of the lateral malleolus and the posterior-superior aspect of the 5th metatarsal styloid process [39]. The peroneal tendons course directly between an imaginary line connecting these easily identified locations with the peroneus brevis located dorsally and the peroneus longus located plantarly. A small linear incision is made through the skin at the center of the imaginary line until the peroneal reti-naculum, with the tendons located within their respective sheaths, has been identified. The sheath to the intended tendon is initially incised in line with the skin incision and protected for later re-approximation after which the peroneal tendon is retrieved through the incision and sharply transected. The foot is then manipulated into inversion and dorsiflexion (if the peroneus brevis has been transected) and the first ray and medial forefoot is manipu-lated into dorsiflexion and inversion (if the peroneus brevis has been trans-ected) to release any adhesions between the peroneal tendons and their respective sheaths and correction assessed. Following release of the peroneal tendon or tendons, the skin edges are re-approximated with a one or two vertical mattress suture of No. 2-0 Nylon incorporating the peroneal tendon sheath and retinaculum into the suture to limit the potential for formation of a tenosynovial fluid leak induced dehiscence or fistula for the reasons described above.

After the soft-tissue contractures described have been assessed and addressed, the osseous alignment of the hindfoot articulations is evaluated. The author has found that the use of a simple intraoperative assessment technique can aid in the determination of the optimal functional alignment of the hindfoot [40]. The technique involves determining the plantar repre-sentation of the subtalar joint axis on the foot by plotting a series of points where no rotation occurs when manual force is applied to the plantar aspect of the foot [41]. Specifically, the examiner uses one thumb to push on the plantar aspect of the foot while the opposite thumb is loading the plantar fifth metatarsal head to detect any resultant supination and/or pronation motions of the foot at the subtalar joint. When the examiner's thumb presses on the plantar foot medial to the subtalar joint axis, then subtalar joint supination will occur. When the examiner's thumb presses lateral to the subtalar joint axis, then subtalar joint pronation will occur. When the examiner's thumb presses directly plantar to the subtalar joint axis, then nei-ther supination nor pronation will occur. This point of no rotation is then marked on the plantar foot. Plotting the points of no rotation, from poste-rior-to-anterior, on the plantar aspect of the foot represents the plantar lo-cation of the subtalar joint axis. The most appropriate subtalar joint axis location is one that is positioned just lateral to the medial calcaneal tubercle at the rearfoot proximally and courses distally through the first metatarsal interspace at the forefoot [41]. Because a prime goal of the surgical correc-tion of unstable hindfoot deformities is to eliminate or reduce excessive extremes of subtalar joint moments during weight-bearing activities, use of this intraoperative assessment technique allows the surgeon to more objectively estimate the location of the subtalar joint axis after surgical cor-rection of the hindfoot complex during surgery [40]. In turn, this allows for better counterbalancing of the subtalar joint pronation and supination moments postoperatively, which helps restore more normal rotational forces acting on the patient's midfoot and forefoot during gait [40,41].

After the subtalar joint axis is mapped out and a supple hindfoot valgus deformity is appreciated, a subtalar arthroeresis is performed to place an oversized subtalar arthroeresis implant within the sinus tarsi (BIOARCH Subtalar Implant System, Wright Medical Technology, Inc., Arlington, Tennessee) [13]. The rationale behind this procedure is based on the goal of hindfoot realignment, which is to align the calcaneus under the mechanical axis of the lower leg. Significant frontal plane deformities are frequently associated with unstable midfoot and hindfoot deformities that are difficult to control [42] and can lead to excessive stress across the midfoot and forefoot causing late collapse of the surgical reconstruction (Fig. 3A) [13]. The use of an oversized subtalar arthroeresis implant is simple to perform, minimally invasive, allows for correction of significant frontal plane deformities about the hindfoot, is reversible, and considerably stiffens the hindfoot allowing protection of the subsequent midfoot and forefoot stabilization procedures [13,42]. The axis of the sinus tarsi is identified by first marking out the lateral malleolus and then identifying and marking the calcaneal-cuboid joint, which is accomplished by first dorsiflexing the foot at the ankle to 90° and carrying an imaginary line from the anterior crest of the tibia to the lateral aspect of the sole of the foot as previously described [43,44]. The lateral aspect of the sinus tarsi is located midway between the distal-anterior tip of the lateral malleolus and the calcaneal-cuboid joint. This location lies between the anterior-lateral portal placement for performing arthroscopy of the subtalar joint and the dorsal-lateral portal for both talar-navicular and calcaneal-cuboid arthroscopy [45–47]. A Steinmann pin is inserted through the skin at the location of the lateral aspect of the sinus tarsi and advanced medially with a slight posterior and plantar angulation until it is felt on the medial side of the foot near the sustentaculum tali inferior to the medial malleolus (Fig. 3B). Verification of the proper location within the sinus tarsi involves several maneuvers. First, the foot is first dorsiflexed and plantarflexed multiple times; and then the hindfoot is inverted and everted multiple times. If the Steinmann pin is truly within the sinus tarsi— and not the ankle joint, which lies in close proximity—the pin will not move with dorsiflexion and plantarflexion because this represents ankle motion and instead, it will move with inversion and eversion of the hindfoot because this represents subtalar motion. Additionally, the use of image intensification will verify proper placement within the sinus tarsi and not the ankle or subtalar joints (Fig. 3C). The Steinmann pin is replaced with the guide wire from the arthroeresis tray and the incision is extended on either side of the initial pin hole to accept the trial implant, which is most commonly 10 mm (Fig. 3D). The trial implant is driven into the sinus tarsi until it is fully seated, which occurs when the implant resides under the talus as verified on an anterior-posterior image intensification view of the foot (Fig. 3E). The alignment of the calcaneus relative to the mechanical axis of the tibia should be assessed and, if the calcaneus continues to be laterally displaced and the subtalar joint axis has failed to become properly aligned,

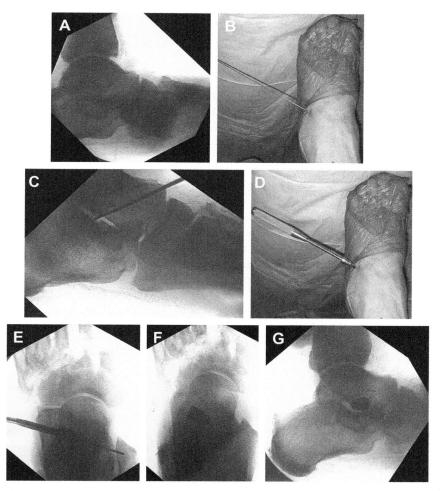

Fig. 3. (*A*) Lateral intraoperative image intensification view of a dislocated Charcot midfoot fracture with associated hindfoot deformity. Anterior-posterior intraoperative clinical (*B*) and lateral image intensification (*C*) views demonstrating proper insertion of the Steinmann pin through the sinus tarsi. Anterior-posterior intraoperative clinical (*D*) and lateral image intensification (*E*) views demonstrating proper insertion of the trial implant through the sinus tarsi. Intraoperative anterior-posterior (*F*) and lateral (*G*) image intensification views demonstrating proper placement of the over-sized subtalar arthroeresis implant within the sinus tarsi, as well as, the complete realignment of the hindfoot that has been achieved.

the trial implant should be removed and the next larger size inserted. This process should be repeated until the calcaneus is directly under the mechanical axis of the lower extremity with a proper subtalar joint axis alignment and little to no hindfoot motion is appreciated with manual stress. After the proper subtalar arthroeresis implant trial size has been verified, the trial implant is removed with care taken to maintain position of the guide wire and the definitive implant is inserted verifying proper alignment and stability as mentioned above (Fig. 3F,G).

If a subtalar arthroeresis cannot be performed secondary to inadequate space within the sinus tarsi to accept the implant, rigid hindfoot valgus deformity, or talar/calcaneal abnormalities such as fracture, erosive or cystic changes, or avascular necrosis (Fig. 4), then a minimum incision arthrodesis of the subtalar joint can be performed. The safe application of minimum incision approaches to the midfoot and hindfoot has been discussed by several authors regarding the performance of arthroscopic débridement and arthrodesis of the subtalar, calcaneal-cuboid, and talar-navicular joints [45–47]. The sinus tarsi is identified in the same fashion as mention above including placement of the Steinmann pin, motion analysis, and image intensification, however, the incision is carried only toward the posterior side of the pin to expose the posterior facet of the subtalar joint (Fig. 5). Under image intensification and 8 mm bone trephine is repeatedly passed through the subtalar joint to resect the articular cartilage and various amounts of the subchondral bone plate. The use of a trephine to prepare joint surfaces for arthrodesis has been safely employed for the tarsometatarsal [13,48] and subtalar, calcaneal-cuboid, and talar-navicular [13,49] joints. Additional resection is performed with the use of a drill, curette and/or small osteotome until resection is deemed adequate. The use of a drill to prepare joint surfaces for arthrodesis has been safely employed in the ankle [50–52] and subtalar joints [52]. The calcaneus is then aligned vertically under the mechanical axis of the lower extremity using the same technique described above and provisional fixation delivered. At times, it can be difficult to maintain ankle and hindfoot alignment while attempting to obtain provisional fixation. A useful technique is to provisionally fixate the ankle with large diameter smooth Steinmann pins with the talus rotated into full dorsiflexion within the ankle mortise before continuing any osseous hindfoot or midfoot surgery (Fig. 6) [53–55]. This technique effectively locks the talus within the ankle mortise in neutral alignment, allowing the surgeon

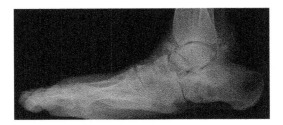

Fig. 4. Weight-bearing lateral radiograph of an acute talar and calcaneal neck fracture in a patient with a series of chronic malaligned Charcot fractures about the midfoot and forefoot. The presence of a fracture within the talus and calcaneus would preclude the use of a subtalar arthroeresis implant and warrant a formal arthrodesis.

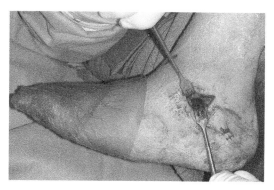

Fig. 5. Intraoperative photograph of the patient shown in Fig. 4 demonstrating the location of and exposure afforded with the minimum incision approach to the posterior facet of the subtalar joint.

to more efficiently and effectively re-align the calcaneus relative to the talus and then the midfoot relative to the hindfoot. The first pin is driven from the anterior-medial border of the distal tibia into the posterior articular surfaces of the ankle. The initial starting point for the first wire begins 5 cm proximal to the distal tip of the medial malleolus and medial to the anterior tibial tendon. The second pin is driven from the posterior-medial border of the distal tibia into the anterior articular surface of the ankle joint. The initial starting

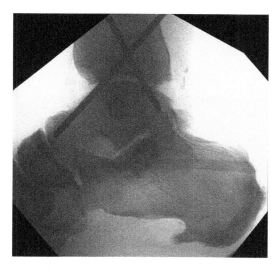

Fig. 6. Lateral intraoperative image intensification view following insertion of crossed Steinmann pins as described in the manuscript to stabilize the ankle which facilitates re-alignment of the midfoot and hindfoot around this stable segment.

point for the second wire begins 5 cm proximal to the distal tip of the medial malleolus and anterior to the posterior tibial tendon. Placing the pins in this manner avoids the saphenous vein and nerve, which course in close proximity to the entry point for both wires [54]. The stability of the fixation is tested by attempting manual dorsiflexion and plantarflexion of the ankle joint, which should be rigid. The pin position is verified with image intensification and when placement is deemed appropriate the pins are bent, cut, and capped to avoid iatrogenic injury and facilitate removal at completion of the surgery. With the ankle stable, the guide wire for an 8.0 mm cannulated titanium screw (Asnis III, Stryker Orthopaedics, Inc., Mahwah, New Jersey) or 7.5 mm cannulated titanium screw (DARCO Headed Screw System; Wright Medical Technology, Inc., Arlington, Tennessee) is then driven from the plantar-posterior aspect of the calcaneus across the posterior aspect of the posterior facet and into the talar body. This positioning corresponds to the location of densely packed bone [56], which enhances fixation, and also resides in a more vertical position outside of the subtalar joint axis, thereby limiting the potential for rotation around the fixation to occur, which would weaken the construct. The appropriate length cannulated screw is then inserted without drilling, tapping, or countersinking in order to have as much contact between the screw and surrounding bone as possible. This is especially important when working with the osteopenic bone frequently encountered in high-risk patients [17,57–59] with long-standing unstable midfoot and hindfoot deformities. The use of a long-thread or fully-threaded pattern screw has the added advantage of capturing the subchondral bone plates and the dense surrounding bone, which limits the potential for late collapse of the arthrodesis site (Fig. 7) [60]. Allogenic bone graft (BioSet IC, RT Allograft Paste, Regeneration Technologies, Inc., Alachua, Florida) and, in especially high-risk patients the addition of FDA off-label, humanitarian use of human recombinant bone morphogenetic

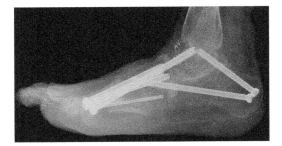

Fig. 7. Lateral radiograph of the same patient shown in Figs. 4 and 5 following multiple re-alignment osteotomies about the forefoot and re-alignment arthrodeses about the midfoot and hindfoot. Note the restoration of near normal pedal alignment and use of long-threaded screws to cross multiple articulations intended to limit potential for collapse as described in the manuscript.

protein-7 (OP-1 Implant; Stryker Orthobiologics, Hopkinton, Massachusetts) impregnated with either autologous platelet rich plasma or autologous bone marrow aspirate that has been percutaneously harvested with a bone marrow aspirate system (Wright Medical Technology, Inc., Arlington, Tennessee) from either the proximal-medial tibia or lateral calcaneus is then packed within the arthrodesis site (Fig. 8). This combination of products exploits the ability to promote osteogenesis, osteoinduction, and osteoconduction across large osseous voids in an immunocompromised host whose host bone is pathologic to begin with and thus, avoids the associated morbidity of autogenous bone graft harvest from either the proximal tibia or iliac crest [33,61–70]. The indications, contraindications, and specific technique for harvesting bone marrow aspirate along with the "pearls for success" advocated and used by the author are published in this issue and will not be repeated here [71]. Intraoperative image intensification and clinical examination are employed to verify adequate alignment of the hindfoot, as well as appropriate fixation and filling of the arthrodesis site. If satisfactory, the surgical site is closed in a single layer using 2-0 Nylon suture and metallic skin staples.

Next, the midfoot and forefoot are manipulated to correct any deformity present [13]. The initial step is to adduct or abduct the forefoot and midfoot into rectus alignment under image intensification (Fig. 9A, B). Next, the forefoot and midfoot are plantarflexed or dorsiflexed on the hindfoot to re-establish a normal metatarsal declination angle (Fig. 9C, D). Finally,

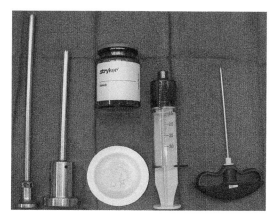

Fig. 8. Instrumentation and products employed to fashion the bone marrow aspirate impregnated allogenic bone graft mixture and resect articulations as described in the manuscript. From left to right: bone trephine plunger, 8 mm round-core biopsy trephine, human recombinant bone morphogenetic protein-7 (*top center*) (OP-1 Implant; Stryker Orthobiologics, Hopkinton, Massachusetts), allogenic bone graft (*bottom center*) (BioSet IC, RT Allograft Paste, Regeneration Technologies, Inc., Alachua, Florida), syringe filled with bone marrow aspirate, and bone marrow aspirate trocar and stylet (Wright Medical Technology, Inc., Arlington, Tennessee).

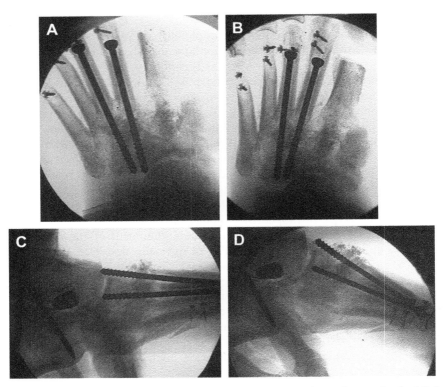

Fig. 9. Anterior-posterior, intraoperative image intensification views of a previously failed Charcot midfoot stabilization demonstrating significant abduction midfoot deformity (*A*) that can be manually reduced to rectus alignment (*B*). Lateral intraoperative image intensification views of the same foot demonstrated in Fig. 9A, B demonstrating significant dorsiflexion midfoot deformity (*C*) that can be manually reduced to rectus alignment (*D*).

the forefoot and midfoot are inverted or everted on the hindfoot to establish a plantigrade forefoot to hindfoot relationship. Occasionally, it is difficult to proceed through these steps without loosing correction and the use of large peri-articular reduction forceps can be especially beneficial. At each step in the reduction the peri-articular reduction, forceps would be strategically placed to maintain reduction so that the next step can be performed (Fig. 10). After clinical examination supports adequate re-alignment of the forefoot and midfoot relative to the hindfoot, then the relationship of the entire foot is assessed under image intensification. After this has been deemed appropriate, minimum incision placement of a large diameter guide wire across the entire medial column is performed (Fig. 11A) [13,72–74]. The most direct approach is to make a small linear incision at the junction between the plantar aspect of the hallux and the weight-bearing surface of the sole of the forefoot. The dissection is carried down to the 1st metatarsal head with gentle blunt dissection and the guide wire for a large diameter

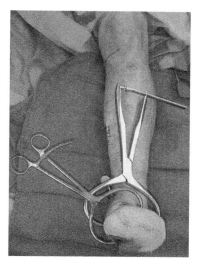

Fig. 10. Intraoperative anterior-posterior view following application of large peri-articular reduction forceps employed to maintain reduction of the midfoot and the realignment demonstrated in Fig. 9. Note the use of provisional ankle stabilization with crossed Steinmann pins during this process.

screw is inserted into the 1st metatarsal head under image intensification and advanced proximally into the talar body. Anterior-posterior and lateral views of the entire foot, as well as anterior-posterior and oblique views of the ankle, will verify proper placement within the contents of the medial column and ensure that inadvertent placement into the medial gutter of the ankle has not occurred, respectively. Once proper placement and alignment is verified under image intensification, a proper length 8.0 mm cannulated titanium screw (Asnis III, Stryker Orthopaedics, Inc., Mahwah, New Jersey) or 7.5 mm cannulated titanium screw (DARCO Headed Screw System; Wright Medical Technology, Inc., Arlington, Tennessee) is then driven across the entire medial column until the head of the screw is seated below the subchondral bone in the 1st metatarsal head and the threads reside within the talar body (Fig. 11B, C). Next, a large diameter guide wire is placed in similar fashion through either the 2nd or 3rd metatarsals into the talar body or the 4th metatarsal into the calcaneus. The 5th metatarsal is rarely "beamed" because some motion about the most lateral aspect of the foot can limit the potential for a rigid and uncompensated varus foot deformity but primarily because the 5th metatarsal itself lies quite lateral to the cuboid and calcaneus, making secure osseous placement difficult, if not impossible. A proper length 6.5 mm cannulated titanium screw (Asnis III, Stryker Orthopaedics, Inc., Mahwah, New Jersey) or 4.3 mm cannulated titanium screw (DARCO Headed Screw System; Wright Medical Technology, Inc., Arlington, Tennessee) is then driven across the aforementioned regions

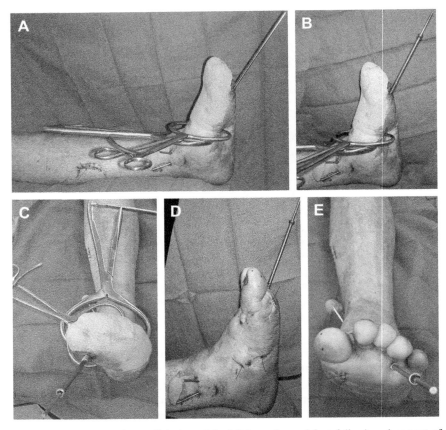

Fig. 11. (*A*) Intraoperative medial view of the left lower leg and foot following placement of large peri-articular reduction clamps about the midfoot and insertion of a large diameter guide wire from the first metatarsal into the talus (ie, medial column "beaming" screw). Intraoperative medial (*B*) and en fass (*C*) views with the appropriate length screw on the guide wire for the medial column. Intraoperative medial (*D*) and en fass (*E*) views with the appropriate length screw on the guide wire extending from the fourth metatarsal into the cuboid (ie, lateral column "beaming" screw). Note the use of provisional ankle stabilization with crossed Steinmann pins during this process.

and seated below the subchondral bone in the respective metatarsal heads (Fig. 11D, E). The provisional Steinmann pin fixation across the ankle is formally removed or, if deemed beneficial in the post-operative period, new Steinmann pins can be placed in extra-articular fashion through the same starting points in the medial distal tibia but extended into the hindfoot and midfoot for more secure fixation as previously described [54,55].

After the osseous alignment has been verified through the use of clinical alignment parameters and intraoperative image intensification, the peri-articular reduction forceps are removed and the involved tarsal-metatarsal and midfoot articulations are identified under image intensification, and minimally invasive incisions are carried directly to the underlying articulations (Fig. 12A). The calcaneal-cuboid joint, talar-navicular joint, and junction space between the calcaneus, talus, navicular, and cuboid can be adequately resected through the sinus tarsi incision using an 8 mm round-core biopsy trephine, drill, curette, and/or osteotome as discussed above. If deemed necessary, the calcaneal-cuboid joint can be formally accessed through the traditional lateral portal used to perform calcaneal-cuboid arthroscopy [45–47] , which is located dorsal to the peroneal tendons and

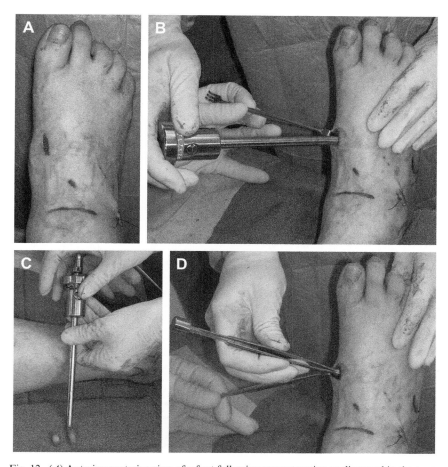

Fig. 12. (A) Anterior-posterior view of a foot following reconstruction as discussed in the manuscript demonstrating the incision placement for access to the first tarsal-metatarsal articulation, which was performed under image intensification. An 8 mm round-core biopsy trephine is being used to resect the articular cartilage on either side of the medial column "beaming" screw discussed in the article (B). Proper technique allows for precise resection of the articulations as demonstrated (C). Following proper joint resection the allogenic bone graft mixture discussed in the manuscript is inserted within the defect (D).

identified based on the topographic landmarks described above [43,44]. Additionally, the talar-navicular joint can be accessed through the traditional dorsal-medial portal used to perform talar-navicular arthroscopy, which is located between the tibialis anterior tendon medially and the extensor hallucis longus tendon laterally [45–47]. An 8 mm round-core biopsy trephine is

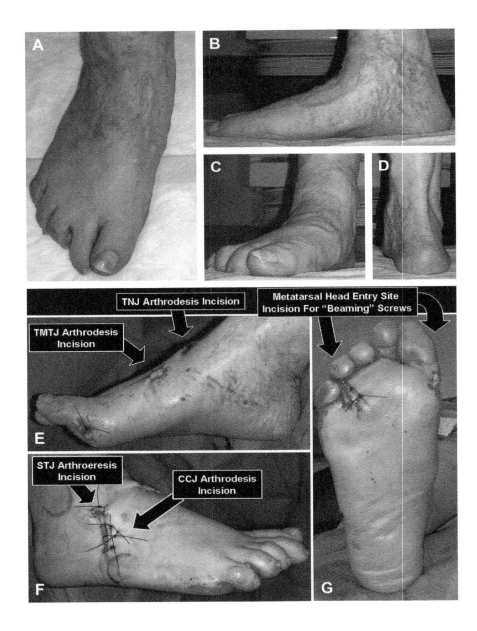

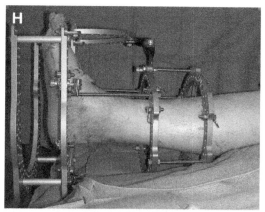

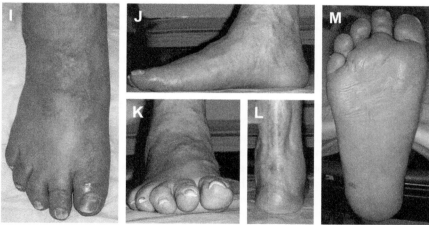

Fig. 13 (*continued*)

Fig. 13. Clinical weight-bearing anterior-posterior (*A*), medial (*B*), en fass (*C*), and hindfoot alignment (*D*) views of a patient with unstable Charcot fracture dislocation about their midfoot that failed conservative treatments. Intraoperative medial (*E*), lateral (*F*), and plantar (*G*) views of the same patient's foot demonstrating the surgical incisions used to perform minimum incision soft-tissue and osseous stabilization as described in the manuscript. This obese patient had dense peripheral neuropathy and failed attempts at preoperative physical therapy gait training and was unable to remain strictly nonweight bearing to her operative side. The use of ring-type external fixation was therefore employed to allow weight sharing on the operative limb for transfers only (*H*). Postoperative, clinical weight-bearing anterior-posterior (*I*), medial (*J*), en fass (*K*), hindfoot alignment (*L*), and plantar (*M*) views of the same patient discussed above, demonstrating a stable and well-aligned foot. Note that additional toe surgery was performed at the time the external fixation device was removed which completed the staged surgical approach employed.

used to core out the articulations on either side of the screw fixation
(Fig. 12B) with care taken to properly expose the subchondral bone plate
and bleeding, healthy cancellous bone (Fig. 12C) [13,48,49]. If any diseased
bone is present following this technique, then the incision should be extended and any nonviable bone resected. The osseous defect is then packed
with a combination of allogenic bone graft (BioSet IC, RT Allograft Paste,
Regeneration Technologies, Inc., Alachua, Florida), human recombinant
bone morphogenic protein-7 (OP-1 Implant; Stryker Orthobiologics, Hopkinton, Massachusetts) impregnated with autologous bone marrow aspirate
as described above (Fig. 12D). The alignment of the entire foot and location
of the hardware is inspected through clinical and image intensification visualization. If satisfactory, the surgical sites are closed in a single layer using
2-0 Nylon suture and metallic skin staples.

A comment should be made regarding the use of intraoperative image intensification as discussed in this manuscript. It is clear that the hazard to the
patient, surgeon, and operating room personnel from exposure, either intermittent or continuous, to the ionizing radiation produced by traditional
C-arm, as well as, mini C-arm or fluoroscopic image intensifiers can be significant [75]. Therefore, it should be clarified that the author uses intraoperative image intensification only in the form of a mini C-arm and only after
performing the topographic analysis discussed above. Furthermore, the mini
C-arm is used to take single snapshots of the surgical field of interest after
properly aligning the foot and ankle to achieve an accurate image with
only rare use of continuous "live" imaging. The benefit of understanding
topography of the foot and ankle and traditional open surgery before under-
taking minimal incision approaches allows the foot and ankle surgeon to
minimize the use of intraoperative image intensification and associated exposure to ionizing radiation through the use of more accurate initial incision
placement to properly perform minimum incision osteotomies and prepare
articular joint surfaces for arthrodesis, as well as proper placement of provisional and permanent internal or external fixation devices.

An external ring fixation system is occasionally employed for those patients who have proven through the use of preoperative physical therapy
consultation to be incapable of remaining strictly nonweight bearing with
regard to the effected limb (Fig. 13) [1,13,17,76]. In this situation the external ring fixation system employed involves the use of a double-stacked foot
plate to allow off-loading of the internal fixation construct, permit weight
sharing during the initial healing phase of 6 to 8 weeks [1,13,17,76], and
allow inspection of the incision sites on a regular basis. An external
bone growth stimulator (Combined Magnetic Field Bone Growth Stimulation, OL 1000 SC Size 3; DONJOY Orthopaedics, LLC, Vista, California)
is universally applied immediately postoperatively and continued on a daily
basis for 6 to 12 months to maximize osseous incorporation [77] and maturation. The rationale is that plain radiographs are notoriously inconclu-
sive when being used to evaluate osseous union and specialized imaging

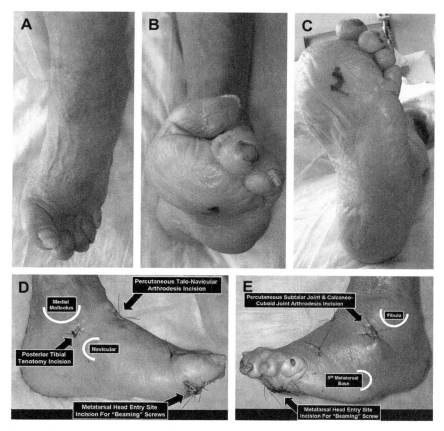

Fig. 14. Clinical nonweight bearing anterior-posterior (*A*), en fass (*B*), and plantar (*C*), views of an elderly, immunocompromised, malnourished, diabetic patient with end stage renal disease on dialysis with a trans-tibial amputation on his contralateral side. The patient had a rigid, non-reducible ankle equinus contracture, cavo-varus foot posture with spasticity from a previously infected lumbar fusion, and multiple forefoot deformities from serial partial metatarsal resections for repeated plantar forefoot ulcerations. He developed a posterior heel ulceration with an attempt at transfer ambulation using a custom-molded ankle-foot orthosis before admission. The patient underwent a percutaneous tendo-Achilles lengthening with percutaneous release of the posterior tibial tendon (*D*) and talar-navicular joint capsule following by revision pan-metatarsal head resection employing a plantar approach, which was followed by a percutaneous triple arthrodesis (*E*) stabilized with medial and lateral column "beaming" screws as discussed in the manuscript. Although the plantar incision required local wound care to heal via secondary intention, anterior-posterior (*F*), en fass (*G*), and plantar (*H*) views demonstrate acceptable re-alignment of his foot and ankle capable of employing a custom-molded shoe with an ankle-foot orthosis. As a result of the surgery, the patient was able to return to community ambulation on a functional limb and prosthesis (*I*).

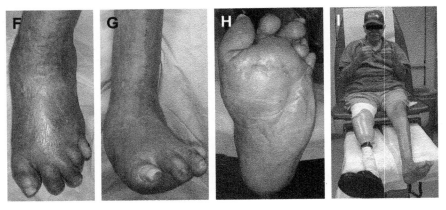

Fig. 14 (*continued*)

techniques, like computerized axial tomography scans, provide limited detail due to the presence of metallic implants. Furthermore, clinical signs of union, such as resolution of edema, warm, and stability of the midfoot and hindfoot to manual stress, are imprecise. Surgical correction of unstable midfoot and hindfoot deformities in the high-risk patient is difficult enough to begin with; however, surgical revision of a previously failed surgical attempt at functional limb salvage is even more challenging, if not impossible. For this reason, the use of multiple forms of technology to enhance osseous incorporation should be employed. If used, the external ring fixation system is removed in the operative theater and a partial weight sharing cast applied for an additional 3 to 4 weeks. If internal fixation alone has been employed a plaster sugar-tong and anterior bolster splint is initially applied until edema has resolved and is followed by application of short-leg nonweight bearing fiberglass casts for 8 to 16 weeks. Gradual conversion to a weight bearing cast, removable walking boot, and finally, custom molded shoe gear and in-shoe orthoses occurs over the ensuing 4 to 6 months time.

Summary

The surgical repair of unstable midfoot and hindfoot deformities in the high-risk patient remains a challenge with little guidance available in the literature. The use of minimally invasive soft-tissue and osseous re-alignment techniques for unstable midfoot and hindfoot deformities in high-risk patients represents a viable alternative to lower limb amputation (Fig. 14). Although the techniques are time-consuming, resource intensive, and have a steep learning curve, the experienced foot and ankle surgeon will find these techniques useful for these difficult limb salvage cases.

References

[1] Zgonis T, Roukis TS, Frykberg RG, et al. Unstable acute and chronic Charcot's deformity: staged skeletal and soft-tissue reconstruction. J Wound Care 2006;15(6):276–80.

[2] Cruz CP, Eidt JF, Capps C, et al. Major lower extremity amputations at a Veterans Affairs hospital. Am J Surg 2003;186(5):449–54.

[3] Pecoraro RE, Reiber GE, Burgess EM. Pathways to diabetic limb amputation. Basis for prevention. Diabetes Care 1990;13(5):513–21.

[4] Trepman E, Nihal A, Pinzur MS. Current topics review: Charcot neuroarthropathy of the foot and ankle. Foot Ankle Int 2005;26(1):46–63.

[5] Shibata T, Tada K, Hashizume C. The results of arthrodesis of the ankle for leprotic neuro-arthropathy. J Bone Joint Surg Am 1990;72(5):749–56.

[6] Simon SR, Tejwani SG, Wilson DL, et al. Arthrodesis as an early alternative to nonoperative management of Charcot arthropathy of the diabetic foot. J Bone Joint Surg Am 2000;82(7): 939–50.

[7] Catanzariti AR, Mendicino R, Haverstock B. Ostectomy for diabetic neuroarthropathy involving the midfoot. J Foot Ankle Surg 2000;39(5):291–300.

[8] Joseph TN, Myerson MS. Correction of multiplanar hindfoot deformity with osteotomy, arthrodesis, and internal fixation. Instr Course Lect 2005;54:269–76.

[9] Bennett GL, Graham CE, Mauldin DM. Triple arthrodesis in adults. Foot Ankle 1991;12(3): 138–43.

[10] Sangeorzan BJ, Smith D, Veith R, et al. Triple arthrodesis using internal fixation in treat-ment of adult foot disorders. Clin Orthop Relat Res 1993;294:299–307.

[11] Sullivan RJ, Aronow MS. Different faces of the triple arthrodesis. Foot Ankle Clin 2002; 7(1):95–106.

[12] Sammarco GJ, Taylor R. Cavovarus foot treated with combined calcaneus and metatarsal osteotomies. Foot Ankle Int 2001;22(1):19–30.

[13] Zgonis T, Roukis TS, Lamm BM. Charcot foot and ankle reconstruction: current thinking and surgical approaches. Clin Podiatr Med Surg 2007;24(2):505–17.

[14] Jeng CL, Vora AM, Myerson MS. The medial approach to triple arthrodesis: indications and technique for management of rigid valgus deformities in high-risk patients. Foot Ankle Clin 2005;10(3):515–21.

[15] Vora AM, Myerson MS. The medial approach to triple arthrodesis: indications and tech-nique for management of rigid valgus deformities in high-risk patients. Techniques in Foot and Ankle Surgery 2005;4(4):258–62.

[16] Bibbo C, Anderson RB, Davis WH. Complications of midfoot and hindfoot athrodesis. Clin Orthop Relat Res 2001;391:45–58.

[17] Roukis TS, Stapleton J, Zgonis T. Addressing psychosocial aspects of care for patients with diabetes undergoing limb salvage surgery. Clin Podiatr Med Surg 2007;24(2):601–10.

[18] Nassar J, Cracchiolo A III. Complications in surgery of the foot and ankle in patients with rheumatoid arthritis. Clin Orthop Relat Res 2001;391:140–52.

[19] Marks RM. Complications of foot and ankle surgery in patients with diabetes. Clin Orthop Relat Res 2001;391:153–61.

[20] Donley BG, Philbin T, Tomford JW, et al. Foot and ankle infections after surgery. Clin Orthop Relat Res 2001;391:162–70.

[21] Acton RK. Surgical principles based on anatomy of the foot: pre-operative planning. Foot Ankle 1982;2(4):200–4.

[22] Sullivan JD. Approaches to the ankle region. Clin Podiatr Med Surg 1986;3(2):289–302.

[23] Attinger CE, Cooper P, Blume P. Vascular anatomy of the foot and ankle. Operative Tech-niques in Plastic and Reconstructive Surgery 1997;4(4):183–98.

[24] Attinger CE, Cooper P, Blume P, et al. The safest surgical incisions and amputations apply-ing the angiosome principles and using the Doppler to assess the arterial-arterial connections of the foot and ankle. Foot Ankle Clin 2001;6(4):745–99.

[25] Attinger CE, Evans KK, Bulan E, et al. Angiosomes of the foot and ankle and clinical implications for limb salvage: reconstruction, incisions, and revascularization. Plast Reconstr Surg 2006;117(Suppl 1):S261–93.
[26] Taylor GI, Palmer JH. The vascular territories (angiosomes) of the body: experimental study and clinical applications. Br J Plast Surg 1987;40(2):113–41, 1987.
[27] Angus PD, Cowell HR. Triple arthrodesis: a critical long-term review. J Bone Joint Surg Br 1986;68(2):260–5.
[28] Graves SC, Mann RA, Graves KO. Triple arthrodesis in older adults. Results after long-term follow-up. J Bone Joint Surg Am 1993;75(3):355–62.
[29] Haritidis JH, Kirkos JM, Provellegios SM, et al. Long-term results of triple arthrodesis: 42 cases followed for 25 years. Foot Ankle Int 1994;15(2):548–51.
[30] Easley ME, Trnka H, Schon LC, et al. Isolate subtalar arthrodesis. J Bone Joint Surg Am 2000;82(5):613–24.
[31] Clain MR, Baxter DE. Simultaneous calcaneal-cuboid and talar-navicular fusion: long-term follow-up study. J Bone Joint Surg Br 1994;76(1):133–6.
[32] Toolan BC, Sangeorzan BJ, Hansen ST Jr. Complex reconstruction for the treatment of dorsolateral peritalar subluxation of the foot: early results after distraction arthrodesis of the calcaneal-cuboid joint in conjunction with stabilization of, and transfer of the flexor digitorum longus tendon to the midfoot to treat acquired pes planovalgus in adults. J Bone Joint Surg Am 1999;81(11):1545–60.
[33] Liporace FA, Bibbo C, Azad A, et al. Bioadjuvants for complex ankle and hindfoot reconstruction. Foot Ankle Clin 2007;12(1):75–106.
[34] Rao SR, Saltzman CL, Wilken J, et al. Increased passive ankle stiffness and reduced dorsiflexion range of motion in individuals with diabetes mellitus. Foot Ankle Int 2006;27(8):617–22.
[35] Nishimoto GS, Attinger CE, Cooper PS. Lengthening the Achilles tendon for the treatment of diabetic plantar forefoot ulceration. Surg Clin North Am 2003;83(3):707–26.
[36] Haro AA, DiDomenico LA. Frontal plane-guided percutaneous tendo Achilles' lengthening. J Foot Ankle Surg. 2007;46(1):55–61.
[37] Schweinberger MH, Roukis TS. Surgical correction of soft-tissue ankle equinus contracture. Clin Podiatr Med Surg 2008;25(4):571–85.
[38] Siegel IM. Equinocavovarus in muscular dystrophy: its treatment by percutaneous tarsal medullostomy and soft tissue release. Arch Surg 1972;104(5):82–4.
[39] Schweinberger MH, Roukis TS. Balancing of the transmetatarsal amputation with peroneus brevis to peroneus longus tendon transfer. J Foot Ankle Surg 2007;46(6):510–4.
[40] Roukis TS, Kirby K. A simple intra-operative technique to align the hindfoot complex. J Am Podiatr Med Assoc 2005;95(5):505–7.
[41] Kirby KA. Subtalar joint axis location and rotational equilibrium theory of foot function. J Am Podiatr Med Assoc 2001;91(9):465–87.
[42] Husain ZS, Fallat LM. Biomechanical analysis of Maxwell-Brancheau arthroeresis implants. J Foot Ankle Surg 2002;41(6):352–8.
[43] Roukis TS. Determining the insertion site for retrograde intramedullary nail fixation of tibiotalocalcaneal arthrodesis: a radiographic and intraoperative anatomical analysis. J Foot Ankle Surg 2006;45(4):227–34.
[44] Roukis TS, Granger D, Zgonis T. A simple technique for performing percutaneous fixation of fifth metatarsal base fractures. J Am Podiatr Med Assoc 2007;97(3):244–5.
[45] Oloff L, Schulhoefer SD, Fanton G, et al. Arthroscopy of the calcaneal-cuboid and talar-navicular joints. J Foot Ankle Surg 1996;35(2):101–8.
[46] Williams MM, Ferkel RD. Subtalar arthroscopy: indications, technique, and results. Arthroscopy 1998;14(4):373–81.
[47] Lui TH. New technique of arthroscopic triple arthrodesis. Arthroscopy 2006;22(4):464 e1–5.
[48] Johnson JE, Johnson KA. Dowel arthrodesis for degenerative arthritis of the tarsometatarsal (Lisfranc) joints. Foot Ankle 1986;6(5):243–53.

[49] Cracchiolo A III, Pearson S, Kitaoka H, et al. Hindfoot arthrodesis in adults utilizing a dowel graft technique. Clin Orthop Relat Res 1990;257:193–203.
[50] Ottolenghi CE, Animoso J, Birgo PH. Percutameous arthrodesis of the ankle joint. Clin Orthop Relat Res 1970;68:72–4.
[51] Graham CE. A new method for arthrodesis of an ankle joint. Clin Orthop Relat Res 1970;68:75–7.
[52] Boer R, Mader K, Pennig D, et al. Tibiotalocalcaneal arthrodesis using a reamed retrograde locking nail. Clin Orthop Relat Res 2007;463:151–6.
[53] Kim DH, Berkowitz MJ, Brunk EF, et al. Technique tip: temporary tibiotalar pinning to facilitate hindfoot arthrodesis. Foot Ankle Int 2007;28(5):645.
[54] Schweinberger MH, Roukis TS. Extra-articular immobilization for protection of percutaneous tendo-Achilles lengthening following transmetatarsal amputation and peripheral arterial bypass surgery. J Foot Ankle Surg 2008.
[55] League AC, Parks BG, Öznur A, et al. Transarticular versus extraarticular ankle pin fixation: a biomechanical study. Foot Ankle Int 2008;29(1):62–5.
[56] Keener BJ, Sizensky JA. The anatomy of the calcaneus and surrounding structures. Foot Ankle Clin 2005;10(3):413–24.
[57] Petrova NL, Foster AV, Edmonds ME. Calcaneal bone mineral density in patients with Charcot neuropathic osteoarthropathy: differences between type 1 and type 2 diabetes. Diabet Med 2005;22(6):756–61.
[58] Hastings MK, Sinacore DR, Fielder FA, et al. Bone mineral density during total contact cast immobilization for a patient with neuropathic (Charcot) arthropathy. Phys Ther 2005;85(3):249–56.
[59] Cheung C. The future of bone healing. Clin Podiatr Med Surg 2005;22(4):631–41.
[60] Hansen ST Jr. Atlas of standard operative techniques: arthrodesis techniques: technique 19-03: subtalar joint arthrodesis with bone block distraction. In: Functional reconstruction of the foot and ankle. Philadelphia: Lippincott Williams & Wilkins; 2000. p. 296–9.
[61] Termaat MF, Den Boer FC, Bakker FC, et al. Current concepts review: bone morphogenetic proteins. J Bone Joint Surg Am 2005;87(6):1367–78.
[62] Toolan BC. Current concepts review: orthobiologics. Foot Ankle Int 2006;27(7):561–6.
[63] Bibbo C, Haskell MD. Recombinant bone morphogenetic protein-2 (rhBMP-2) in high-risk foot and ankle surgery: surgical techniques and preliminary results of a prospective, intention-to-treat study. Techniques in Foot and Ankle Surgery 2007;6(2):71–9.
[64] Roukis TS, Zgonis T, Tiernan B. Autologous platelet-rich plasma in wound and bone graft healing: a review of the literature and commercially available products. Adv Ther 2006;23(2):218–37.
[65] Bibbo C, Bono CM, Lin SS. Union rates using autologous platelet rich concentrate alone and with bone graft in high-risk foot and ankle surgery. J Surg Orthop Adv 2005;14(1):17–22.
[66] Gandhi A, Bibbo C, Pinzur M, et al. The role of platelet-rich plasma in foot and ankle surgery. Foot Ankle Clin 2005;10(4):621–37.
[67] Barnett MD Jr, Pomeroy GC. Use of platelet-rich plasma and bone marrow-derived mesenchymal stem cells in foot and ankle surgery. Techniques in Foot and Ankle Surgery 2007;6(2):89–94.
[68] Yamaguchi Y, Kubo T, Murakami T, et al. Bone marrow cells differentiate into wound myofibroblasts and accelerate the healing of wounds with exposed bones when combined with an occlusive dressing. Br J Dermatol 2005;152(4):616–27.
[69] Hernigou PH, Mathieu G, Poignard A, et al. Percutaneous autologous bone-marrow grafting for nonunions: surgical technique. J Bone Joint Surg Am 2006;88(Supp 1):322–7.
[70] Schweinberger MH, Roukis TS. Percutaneous autologous bone-marrow harvest from the calcaneus and proximal tibia: surgical technique. J Foot Ankle Surg 2007;46(5):411–4.
[71] Schade VL, Roukis TS. Percutaneous bone marrow aspirate and bone graft harvesting techniques in the lower extremity. Clin Podiatr Med Surg 2008;25(4):733–42.

[72] Grant WP, Sullivan RW. Medial column rodding for correction of the Charcot foot. In: Programs and abstracts of the American College of Foot and Ankle Surgeons 55th Annual Meeting and Scientific Seminar. Palm Springs, 1997. p. 13.

[73] Grant WP, Jerlin EA, Pietrzak WS, et al. The utilization of autologous growth factors for the facilitation of fusion in complex neuropathic fractures in the diabetic population. Clin Podiatr Med Surg 2005;22(4):561–84.

[74] Sammarco GJ, Guioa RG. Treatment of Charcot midfoot collapse with transverse midtarsal arthrodesis fixed with multiple long intramedullary screws. In: Programs and abstracts of the Australian Orthopaedic Association. Adelaide (Australia): 2003 Referenced in J Bone Joint Surg Br 2004;86(Suppl 4):477.

[75] Shoaib A, Rethnam U, Bansal R, et al. A comparison of radiation exposure with conventional versus mini C-arm in orthopedic extremity surgery. Foot Ankle Int 2008;29(1):58–61.

[76] Roukis TS, Zgonis T. Post-operative shoe modifications for weightbearing with the Ilizarov external fixation system. J Foot Ankle Surg 2004;43(6):433–5.

[77] Petrisor B, Lau JT. Electrical bone stimulation: an overview and its use in high-risk and Charcot foot and ankle reconstructions. Foot Ankle Clin 2005;10(4):609–20.

CLINICS IN
PODIATRIC
MEDICINE AND
SURGERY

Clin Podiatr Med Surg
25 (2008) 681–690

Corrective Midfoot Osteotomies

John J. Stapleton, DPM, AACFAS[a,b],
Lawrence A. DiDomenico, DPM, FACFAS[c],
Thomas Zgonis, DPM, FACFAS[d,*]

[a]*Foot and Ankle Surgery, VSAS Orthopaedics, Lehigh Valley Hospital, Cedar Crest Campus, Allentown, PA, USA*
[b]*Penn State College of Medicine, 500 University Drive, Hershey, PA 17033, USA*
[c]*Ankle and Foot Care Center, 8175 Market Street, Boardman, OH 44512, USA*
[d]*Department of Orthopaedics/Podiatry Division, The University of Texas Health Science Center at San Antonio, 7703 Floyd Curl Drive (MSC 7776), San Antonio, TX 78229, USA*

Corrective osteotomies about the midfoot are indicated for angular and rotational deformities. Appropriate positioning of the osseous segments following midfoot osteotomy is challenging because of influential forces around the hindfoot/ankle and the forefoot that must be considered. Initially, midfoot osteotomies were reserved for the correction of the severe rigid pes cavus foot [1]. Currently, surgeons have used angular, rotational, and translational deformity corrections that can be achieved through the midfoot, expanding the indications for an osteotomy through this region of the foot [2–4]. In addition, midfoot osteotomies often avoid the extensive soft tissue exposure required for multiple joint arthrodesis procedures because these procedures can be performed through minimum or percutaneous incisions [5]. Typical indications for a midfoot osteotomy are rigid pes cavus, talipes equinus-varus, rigid metatarsus adductus, malunions associated with midfoot or rearfoot arthrodesis, and Charcot neuro-osteoarthropathy midfoot deformities [1,3,4,6–11].

The goal of a corrective midfoot osteotomy is to re-establish a plantigrade foot during stance, which implies that the first metatarsal head, fifth metatarsal head, and calcaneus are on the same plane during stance. Limited normal parameters exist for performing midfoot osteotomies and it is therefore imperative that the surgeon have detailed knowledge and sound understanding of all compensatory joint motions that exist proximal and distal to the intended osteotomy to achieve successful deformity correction through the midfoot.

---

* Corresponding author.
E-mail address: zgonis@uthscsa.edu (T. Zgonis).

0891-8422/08/$ - see front matter © 2008 Elsevier Inc. All rights reserved.
doi:10.1016/j.cpm.2008.05.004 *podiatric.theclinics.com*

Physical examination

The physical examination must be systematic and should include evalua-tion of the entire lower extremity when non–weight bearing, during stance, and while ambulating. Emphasis is placed on identifying the apex of the deformity and compensatory motion or joint contractures that are present. Deformity should be evaluated in regards to its length, angulation, rotation, and translation. In the foot, particularly in the midfoot region, this evalua-tion can become challenging because of the short osseous segments and mul-tiple articulations proximally and distally. For this reason, it is important to establish clinical parameters and to correlate those findings with the neces-sary radiographs to provide an adequate description of the deformity to be corrected. The contralateral extremity, if unaffected, facilitates the examina-tion and serves as an internal control for the patient. The surgeon must eval-uate the deformity in the frontal, sagittal, and transverse planes to plan adequately the necessary osteotomy, realignment, and adjunctive proce-dures that may be required to restore a plantigrade foot. Radiographs are obtained to evaluate the deformity and to create reference lines to facilitate precise surgical planning. Weight-bearing anterior-posterior and lateral radiographs of the lower leg, ankle, and foot, along with a hindfoot align-ment view, must be obtained and correlated with the clinical examination. The importance of weight-bearing radiographs for the evaluation of the deformity cannot be overstated because subtle deformities not readily ap-parent on clinical examination become easily detected. If the patient's weight-bearing lower leg radiographs demonstrate proximal deformity or limb–length discrepancy, then weight-bearing anterior-posterior and lateral mechanical axis radiographs should be obtained from the hip to the ankle. The mechanical axis is a line drawn from the center of the femoral head to the center of the ankle joint. If the mechanical axis deviates more than 1 cm from the center of the knee joint, then a deformity proximal to the ankle is located in the tibia or femur. Understanding the influence of supra-pedal structural deformities is paramount, particularly when these supra-pedal structural deformities exceed the range of motion that is present in compen-satory joints about the foot and ankle. For example, a varus deformity of the tibia can lead to fixed subtalar joint inversion and compensatory fore-foot valgus. Conversely, a valgus deformity of the tibia can lead to fixed sub-talar joint eversion and compensatory forefoot varus. The development of these foot and ankle deformities from proximal deformities of the tibia and femur depend on the compensatory range of motion throughout the foot and ankle. At times, these deformities may require osteotomies of the rearfoot/ankle, tibia, or femur, in addition to the midfoot, to achieve the desired correction.

Position of the forefoot and the rearfoot is paramount in planning for a midfoot osteotomy. The surgeon should examine rearfoot position when non–weight bearing and during stance. It should be determined if forefoot position is influencing rearfoot deformity and vice versa. The forefoot should be plantigrade, allowing for equal transfer of weight throughout the foot. Forefoot varus produces increased weight transfer to the lateral border of the foot and may cause a compensatory calcaneal valgus deformity. Conversely, forefoot valgus deformities produce increased weight transfer to the medial border of the foot and may cause a compensatory calcaneal varus deformity. Deformities about the forefoot can usually be corrected with midfoot osteotomies. Forefoot varus and valgus are usually corrected through rotation of the forefoot segment following midfoot osteotomy. Sagittal and transverse plane forefoot deformities can be corrected with wedge-based midfoot osteotomies and translation, respectively. However, an attempt to correct noncompensatory deformities and fixed compensatory deformities about the rearfoot, particularly the calcaneus and subtalar joint, with midfoot osteotomies should not be attempted. A calcaneal osteotomy or subtalar joint arthrodesis, in addition to a corrective midfoot osteotomy, is needed for these associated rearfoot deformities [6]. Correction through the midfoot will not correct a rearfoot deformity unless the deformity was compensatory to the deformed forefoot position and joint contracture has not developed. An example would be a fixed forefoot varus with a compensatory heel valgus. When a block is placed preoperatively under the forefoot, the calcaneus inverts from its valgus position, resuming a neutral position. In this case scenario, a midfoot osteotomy to correct the fixed forefoot varus will simultaneously correct the calcaneal valgus that was compensatory with no evidence of subtalar joint contracture.

Sagittal plane deformities in the pes cavus foot are a frequent indication for a midfoot osteotomy [1,7,11]. The osteotomy is designed with a dorsally based wedge to dorsiflex the forefoot and decrease the arch height [1,7,11]. At times, a wedge osteotomy has to be taken from the navicular-cuneiform joint extending into the cuboid to obtain adequate correction. Anterior equinus of the forefoot can be corrected with a midfoot dorsally based wedge osteotomy. Procurvatum deformities and ankle equinus cannot be corrected with a midfoot osteotomy, and additional soft tissue or osseous procedures about the ankle are required. It is important to evaluate the ankle on lateral weight-bearing radiographs for procurvatum and recurvatum deformities of the ankle. At times, dorsiflexory stress radiographs are indicated to ensure an anterior osseous impingement is not evident at the ankle and that sufficient ankle joint dorsiflexion remains when considering correction of an anterior equinus by way of a midfoot osteotomy. In addition, posterior osseous cavus deformities should be corrected with calcaneal osteotomies, as opposed to midfoot osteotomies [6,9]. Plantar-based midfoot wedge osteotomies can be used to correct a Charcot midfoot deformity [8]. The authors have found that a midfoot osteotomy in a Charcot foot is best performed if complete consolidation and stability exist about the midfoot [12–14]. The clinical scenario in which a midfoot osteotomy would be indicated for a Charcot foot is one with a plantar midfoot ulcer as a result of a rigid, stable, "rocker-bottom" deformity [13,14]. If instability persists, a midfoot osteotomy should be avoided and an extended joint arthrodesis should be considered instead [13,14].

Rotational alignment should be determined and quantified. Radiographs to measure rotation are difficult and not routinely used. Clinical examination is used to determine the presence and degree of rotational malalignment. With the patient seated, the knee is flexed at 90°, the patellar tubercle is placed directly anterior, and the malleoli position is obtained and assessed for rotational deformity. At this point, a line drawn along the anterior tibial crest is made and the bisection should be aligned with the second metatarsal. The degree of internal (ie, abduction) and external (ie, adduction) rotation is then quantified using a goniometer. In difficult cases with marked rotation and suspected proximal deformity, it may be necessary to obtain computerized axial tomography of the hip, distal femur, proximal tibia, and ankle malleoli to define the rotational deformity more accurately.

Evaluation of joint range of motion is paramount and cannot be overlooked. Flexibility of the foot is determined. Compensatory rigid joint contractures, particularly of the subtalar joint, need to be determined. In addition, hypermobility and joint laxity of the first ray are considered relative contraindications for performing a midfoot osteotomy unless they are addressed. Soft tissue contractures should be evaluated and adjunctive soft tissue releases performed in conjunction with the midfoot osteotomy [15]. A good example is the release of the plantar fascia in conjunction with a midfoot osteotomy for the correction of a semirigid pes cavus foot [1,15]. The surgeon must also consider tendon balancing of the foot to determine if a tendon transfer should be performed. In the paralytic foot with deformity, tendon transfers are often necessary, in addition to osseous deformity correction, to improve function and establish a plantigrade foot [15].

Corrective midfoot osteotomies: surgical technique

The surgical technique for a midfoot osteotomy begins with the patient under general anesthesia and fully paralyzed. A popliteal block can be placed preoperatively for postoperative analgesia. The leg should be directly supine, avoiding any internal or external rotation. In addition, it is imperative to have the entire foot, ankle, and lower leg fully prepped and draped to allow evaluation of the alignment of the foot, ankle, and lower leg intraoperatively. Any concomitant procedures to the hindfoot, ankle, or tibia for deformity correction should be performed before the midfoot osteotomy, starting with the most proximal deformity and working distally. If functional tendon transfers are required, the authors prefer to delay the tendon transfer until clinical and radiographic healing of the osteotomy is complete. The rationale for staging the tendon transfer is to avoid delay of the rehabilitation phase that is required early in the postoperative period for a successful functional tendon transfer. Typically, range of motion for a functional tendon transfer begins at 3 weeks and muscle strengthening at 6 weeks, which cannot be accomplished if the tendon transfers have been performed concomitantly with an osteotomy because the immobilization period for healing of the osteotomy is generally 10 to 12 weeks.

Osteotomy techniques for the midfoot vary according to the deformity present. Osteotomies can be performed through four percutaneous incisions or through two or more minimum incisions. Rotational and translational deformities can be corrected through a percutaneous osteotomy placed over the central aspect of the cuneiforms and cuboid. The osteotomy should never be placed along the metatarsal bases or along the tarsal-metatarsal joint, even if a previous tarsal-metatarsal joint arthrodesis was performed. An osteotomy that passes in this direction will cause vascular injury to the distal perforating arteries in the intermetatarsal spaces. A Gigli saw can be used through appropriately placed percutaneous incisions. If wedge osteotomies are necessary to correct the deformity, the authors use two minimum incisions placed medially and laterally, which allow precise wedge resection and removal of the osseous wedge, and ensure appropriate positioning of the two segments to achieve the desired correction. Regardless of the osteotomy technique, the goals are to protect the neurovascular bundle, preserve the periosteal blood supply, and minimize thermal necrosis [1,7,16].

Percutaneous Gigli saw technique for an osteotomy of the midfoot is performed through four percutaneous incisions. The incisions are placed dorsal-medial, dorsal-lateral, plantar-lateral, and plantar-medial. The incisions are made directly to bone, avoiding injury to the neurovascular bundle and tendon structures. A periosteal elevator is then used to create a tunnel deep to the soft tissue structures dorsally and plantarly. Periosteal stripping is minimized and only created over the path of the osteotomy. The location of the incisions should be confirmed with intraoperative image intensification. In addition, Kirchner wires can be inserted medially and laterally in the path of the planned osteotomy. This technique provides a cutting guide for the Gigli saw. The Gigli saw is first passed plantarly, then dorsally, with the use of a large hemostat to facilitate transfer from one incision to the next. This procedure can be performed without a tourniquet to ensure the neurovascular bundle is not transected. The osteotomy should not be performed from dorsal to plantar or plantar to dorsal because this can lead to neurovascular injury. Typically, the osteotomy is performed from medial to lateral but can be performed cautiously from lateral to medial (Fig. 1).

Incision placement is paramount in performing the osteotomy through two limited incisions and cannot be overlooked. A 3-cm skin incision is made dorsal-medial over the medial cuneiform and extends proximal to the navicular-cuneiform joint and distal to insertion of the tibialis anterior tendon. It is not necessary to carry the incision distally to the first metatarsal-cuneiform joint or to transect the tibialis anterior tendon. This incision should be placed just proximal and inferior to the anterior tibial tendon and distal and dorsal to the insertion of the posterior tibial tendon. The

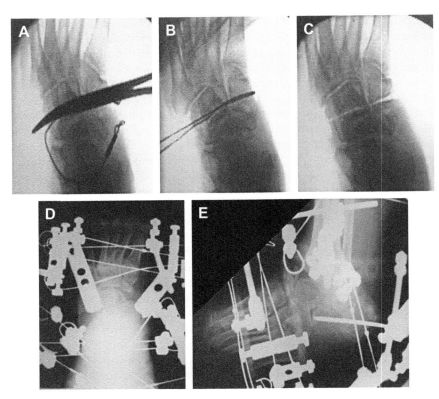

Fig. 1. (*A*) Intraoperative image intensification anterior-posterior view demonstrating proper passing of the Gigli saw through four percutaneous incisions. Intraoperative image intensification anterior-posterior view before (*B*) and following (*C*) completion of the midfoot osteotomy. Postoperative non–weight-bearing anterior-posterior (*D*) and lateral (*E*) radiographs demonstrating realignment of the forefoot following corrective midfoot osteotomy fixated with a ring-type external fixation device.

lateral incision is 3 cm in length and is placed on the dorsal-lateral aspect of the cuboid, just dorsal to the peroneal brevis and longus tendon and plantar to the peroneus tertius tendon. The incision is placed beginning just distal to the calcaneal-cuboid joint and extends to the fourth and fifth metatarsal bases as they articulate with the cuboid. Caution should be used to avoid placing the lateral incision too plantar because this placement creates difficult exposure of the cuboid and retraction of the peroneal tendons. Arthrotomy and transection of the joints surrounding the osteotomy medially and laterally should not be performed; instead, an 18-gauge needle can be placed to identify the location of the joint, if needed. Ligament structures to these joints should be preserved to accomplish deformity correction after appropriate positioning of the osteotomy. A midfoot osteotomy using two minimum incisions is performed initially with a sagittal saw and then completed with an osteotome or flexible chisel. Kirchner wires are again placed with intraoperative image intensification to serve as a guide for the wedge resection and to serve as an osteotomy guide. In addition, hash marks are made perpendicular to the planned osteotomy with a small sagittal saw blade or electrocautery. This technique is advantageous in establishing orientation of the proximal and distal segments after the osteotomy is completed. The use of a sagittal saw is to establish the orientation of the planned osteotomy. Hand instrumentation, such as an osteotome, should be used to prevent thermal necrosis associated with the use of power instrumentation [16]. A narrow osteotome or flexible chisel should be used to prevent fracture propagation perpendicular to the osteotomy. After the osteotomy is performed, it is loosened with an osteotome, a smooth lamina spreader is inserted, and the osteotomy is distracted for 3 to 5 minutes to relax the surrounding soft tissues. Distraction in this manner mobilizes the distal segment, facilitating positioning and deformity correction. In addition, for wedge-based osteotomies, it is advantageous to maintain a periosteal hinge at the apex of the wedge to facilitate closure (Fig. 2).

After the osteotomy is performed and placed in the desired position, it can be fixated with internal fixation, external fixation, or a combination of both. The authors have found it advantageous to stabilize the osteotomy with Steinmann pins if external fixation is used, or guide wires for cannulated screws if internal fixation is to be used, to allow assessment of the desired position before definitive fixation. A metallic instrument cover is typically used to simulate weight bearing to ensure a plantigrade foot is obtained intraoperatively. Circular ring-type external fixation is advantageous in the presence of severe deformities requiring gradual corrections, osteopenia, Charcot neuro-osteoarthropathy, and neuromuscular deformities, and in patients who require early weight bearing [5,12,14,17,18].

Postoperatively, admission with in-patient observation is necessary for 24 hours for pain management and neurovascular monitoring. If internal fixation was used, the patient is initially placed in a bulky, well-padded dressing from toes to knee and a sugar-tong plaster splint for immobilization until edema has subsided. Patients who have external fixation are treated with weekly dressing changes and inspection of the pin sites. Initial radiographs are taken at 2 weeks, followed by gradual removal of all skin sutures and metallic staples.

Patients who have external fixation may be permitted to weight share with a modified shoe after suture removal at 2 weeks if peripheral sensory neuropathy is not present [19]. Patients who have internal fixation are maintained non–weight bearing until radiographic evidence of healing is evident, usually at 6 to 8 weeks postoperative. At that time, a short leg, weight-bearing cast is applied for 2 weeks, followed by a removable walking boot, until complete clinical and radiographic healing is apparent, generally at 10 to 12 weeks postoperative. The patient is then placed into extradepth shoe gear with in-shoe accommodative orthoses or brace therapy, as indicated for life.

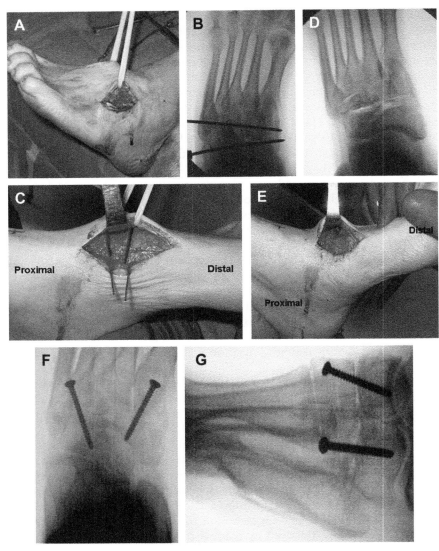

Fig. 2. (*A*) Intraoperative lateral photograph following subperiosteal dissection with a two-incision approach to the midfoot. Note the use of a rubber drain to elevate and protect the dorsal soft tissues and neurovascular structures. Intraoperative image intensification anterior-poster (*B*) and medial photograph (*C*) of the same foot demonstrating use of medial-to-lateral Kirschner wires as an osteotomy guide. Note the precise osteotomies that have been created to perform a dorsiflexory-abductory wedge osteotomy. Intraoperative image intensification anterior-posterior (*D*) and medial photograph (*E*) following removal of the osseous wedge demonstrating multiplanar deformity correction. Intraoperative image intensification anterior-posterior (*F*) and lateral (*G*) radiographs following placement of internal fixation to stabilize the corrective midfoot osteotomy.

Patients who have Charcot neuro-osteoarthropathy deformities who undergo a midfoot osteotomy are not permitted weight bearing, regardless of the method of fixation used. These patients are kept non–weight bearing until radiographic healing and then 50% longer to ensure complete osseous incorporation before transitioning into a weight-bearing cast or removable walking boot. In addition, total contact casts are preferable to walking boots in this patient population, to minimize torque on the osteotomy while initial weight bearing is permitted, generally at 4 to 6 weeks following removal of the external fixation device. A removable walking boot is then continued until clinical and radiographic evidence of healing is complete.

Complications

Soft tissue complications are usually associated with severe deformities, vascular insufficiency, or previously traumatized tissues. Corrections that place excessive tension on the soft tissue envelope and the neurovascular structures can lead to significant complications. These patients should be corrected gradually over a period of time using a ring-type external fixation system that limits the potential to develop skin necrosis and neurovascular insult.

Delayed unions and nonunions are rare but can occur, particularly in high-risk patients, such as those who have diabetes or Charcot neuroarthropathy, those who abuse tobacco or use corticosteroids, or those who have avascular bone associated with previous trauma. These patients may benefit from judicious use of orthobiologic technology and bone growth stimulation to facilitate primary osseous healing.

Malunion often occurs from inadequate preoperative planning, poor intraoperative positioning, or early weight bearing. Attention to detail during the preoperative physical examination is paramount in understanding associated deformities, joint contractures, and compensatory motion proximal and distal to the osteotomy to prevent malunion and resultant deformity. In addition, time spent intraoperatively to ensure appropriate osteotomy placement and positioning cannot be overstated. Postoperative transition to full weight bearing should not occur until radiographic healing is evident, unless an external fixator is used to prevent motion across the osteotomy.

Summary

Corrective midfoot osteotomies represent an effective surgery to treat select pedal deformities. Knowledge of deformity planning and normal anatomic relationships is important to allow foot and ankle surgeons to achieve their goal of re-establishing a plantigrade foot capable of withstanding the repetitive stress associated with ambulation. Percutaneous or minimum incision surgical techniques to realign the midfoot in the high-risk patient are master level techniques that require extensive surgical experience and detailed knowledge of lower extremity biomechanics.

References

[1] Groner TW, DiDomenico LA. Midfoot osteotomies for the cavus foot. Clin Podiatr Med Surg 2005;22(2):247–64.

[2] Dehne R. Osteotomy in the pediatric foot. Foot Ankle Clin 2001;6(3):599–614.

[3] Gordon JE, Luhmann SJ, Dobbs MB, et al. Combined midfoot osteotomy for severe fore-foot adductus. J Pediatr Orthop 2003;23(1):74–8.

[4] Harley BD, Fritzhand AJ, Little JM, et al. Abductory midfoot osteotomy procedure for metatarsus adductus. J Foot Ankle Surg 1995;34(2):153–62.

[5] Paley D. The correction of complex foot deformities using Ilizarov's distraction osteotomies. Clin Orthop Relat Res 1993;293:97–111.

[6] Dierauer S, Schafer D, Hefti F. Osteotomies of the mid- and back-foot in recurrent club foot. Orthopade 1999;28(2):117–24.

[7] Conti SF, Kirchner JS, VanSickle D. Midfoot osteotomies. Foot Ankle Clin 2001;6(3): 519–32.

[8] Myerson MS, Henderson MR, Saxby T, et al. Management of midfoot diabetic neuroarthropathy. Foot Ankle Int 1994;15(5):233–41.

[9] Sammarco GJ, Taylor R. Cavovarus foot treated with combined calcaneus and metatarsal osteotomies. Foot Ankle Int 2001;22(1):19–30.

[10] Toolan BC. Revision of failed triple arthrodesis with an opening-closing wedge osteotomy of the midfoot. Foot Ankle Int 2004;25(7):456–61.

[11] Tullis BL, Mendicino RW, Catanzariti AR, et al. The Cole midfoot osteotomy: a retrospective review of 11 procedures in 8 patients. J Foot Ankle Surg 2004;43(3):160–5.

[12] Jolly GP, Zgonis T, Polyzois V. External fixation in the management of Charcot neuroarthropathy. Clin Podiatr Med Surg 2003;20(4):741–56.

[13] Zgonis T, Roukis TS, Frykberg RG, et al. Unstable acute and chronic Charcot's deformity: staged skeletal and soft-tissue reconstruction. J Wound Care 2006;15(6):276–80.

[14] Zgonis T, Roukis TS, Lamm BM. Charcot foot and ankle reconstruction: current thinking and surgical approaches. Clin Podiatr Med Surg 2007;24(3):505–17.

[15] David A, Tiemann A, Richter J, et al. [Corrective soft tissue interventions for equinovarus deformity. Foot deformities after tibial compartment syndrome]. Unfallchirurg 1997; 100(5):371–4 [in German].

[16] Roukis TS. Corrective ankle osteotomies. Clin Podiatr Med Surg 2004;21(3):353–70.

[17] Koczewski P, Shadi M, Napiontek M. Foot lengthening using the Ilizarov device: the transverse tarsal joint resection versus osteotomy. J Pediatr Orthop 2002;11(1):68–72.

[18] Zgonis T, Jolly GP, Blume P. External fixation use in arthrodesis of the foot and ankle. Clin Podiatr Med Surg 2004;21(1):1–15.

[19] Roukis TS, Zgonis T. Postoperative shoe modifications for weightbearing with the Ilizarov external fixation system. J Foot Ankle Surg 2004;43(6):433–5.

ELSEVIER
SAUNDERS

Clin Podiatr Med Surg
25 (2008) 691–719

CLINICS IN
PODIATRIC
MEDICINE AND
SURGERY

Percutaneous Fixation of Forefoot, Midfoot, Hindfoot, and Ankle Fracture Dislocations

Jeffrey R. Baker, DPM, AACFAS[a,b,*],
Jason P. Glover, DPM[c], Patrick A. McEneaney, DPM[b]

[a]Weil Foot and Ankle Institute, 1455 Gold Road, Suite 110, Des Plaines, IL 60610, USA
[b]Podiatric Medicine and Surgery–36 Residency, Weiss Memorial Hospital Podiatric Surgical
Residency Program, 4646 N. Marine Drive, Chicago, IL 60640, USA
[c]Rutherford Orthopaedics, 139 Doctor Henry Norris Drive, Rutherfordton, NC 28139, USA

Foot and ankle trauma is a challenging injury subset encountered by the foot and ankle surgeon. An understanding of the intricacies involved in the treatment of foot and ankle trauma is paramount before initiating care in complex patients such as the high-risk patient. The complex nature of foot and ankle trauma is magnified when seen in the high-risk patient. Padnalium and Donely [1] described five major categories of high-risk foot and ankle patients, which included (1) diabetes; (2) tobacco use; (3) peripheral vascular disease; (4) traumatic injury; and (5) malnutrition. Also cited were alcoholism, corticosteroid use, and poor compliance with medical instructions as additional factors classifying a patient as a high-risk foot and ankle patient [1].

The management of traumatic injuries in the high-risk patient has several objectives, based on the structure and function of the foot and ankle. These objectives include preservation of neurovascular status, preservation of the plantar skin and fat pad, maintenance of a plantigrade foot, osseous union of fracture fragments, and prevention of infection [2].

Foot and ankle trauma encompasses two types of injury: osseous injury and soft tissue injury. Both a fracture and a dislocation have the potential to compromise the soft tissue envelope and significantly increase the severity of the traumatic injury to the foot and ankle [1–12] because the soft tissue

* Corresponding author. Weil Foot and Ankle Institute, 1455 Gold Road, Suite 110, Des Plaines, IL 60610.
E-mail address: jrb@weil4feet.com (J.R. Baker).

0891-8422/08/$ - see front matter © 2008 Elsevier Inc. All rights reserved.
doi:10.1016/j.cpm.2008.05.003

envelope of the foot and ankle is thin, which increases the potential for soft tissue compromise with trauma to the foot and ankle [1,7]. Therefore, careful handling and preservation of the soft tissue envelope is of paramount importance. With a stable soft tissue envelope, the potential for underlying osseous healing is improved and the complication rate reduced [12].

Open reduction internal fixation is the standard surgical management method for traumatic osseous injury to the foot and ankle. Because of the potential for dehiscence and infection with this technique, less invasive procedures for osseous stabilization, such as percutaneous fixation, have been described [3–5,7–12]. Percutaneous fixation is a minimally invasive technique for osseous stabilization of fractures and dislocations [3–5,7–12]. This technique is characterized by the use of small incisions for insertion of rigid internal fixation with minimal soft tissue dissection, to achieve osseous stability with the assistance of intraoperative image intensification [3–5,7–12]. Using this technique minimizes potential damage to the vascular supply and reduces the incidence of osseous infection [5]. The major disadvantages of percutaneous fixation techniques are the potential for less than optimal reduction due to the lack of direct visualization of the osseous injury and their technically demanding nature [5,12]. However, in experienced hands, percutaneous fixation for foot and ankle trauma in the high-risk patient is a safe and satisfactory method of osseous stabilization without increased physical strain on the patient. This article provides an overview of percutaneous surgical fixation methods and their role in foot and ankle trauma for the high-risk patient.

Phalanx fractures

Several types of fracture patterns are seen in phalanx fractures. If the mechanism of injury can be identified, then it can aid in reduction and treatment. Transverse plane injuries typically are a result of an abduction-adduction force that causes a spiral oblique or transverse fracture [13]. An example commonly seen is when a patient hits his/her fifth toe on bedroom furniture while walking in the dark. Sagittal plane injuries result from a direct compaction, hyperflexion, or hyperextension injury. Frontal plane injuries are usually due to a rotational or inversion-eversion force. Phalanx injuries are infrequent and are usually components of transverse or sagittal plane mechanisms.

Most phalanx fractures are minimally displaced and are often successfully treated with "buddy splinting" to an adjacent digit with protected weight bearing in a supportive athletic or surgical shoe. The fracture usually heals uneventfully within 4 to 6 weeks.

Under certain conditions, fixation needs to be considered. In the high-risk patient, if more than one third of the articular surface is involved or if displacement is more than 2 to 3 mm, the authors recommend percutaneous surgical fixation. The authors prefer this technique to decrease the possibility of nonunion with phalanx fractures in the high-risk patient, which can lead to osseous prominences, hyperkeratotic lesions, and ulceration (Fig. 1).

Metatarsal fractures

Metatarsal fractures account for 35% of all foot fractures and 5% of total skeletal fractures [14]. Closed reduction may be attempted, to restore appropriate length and to reduce rotational malalignments but often, closed treatment alone is not sufficient to maintain alignment. If an anatomic relationship can be achieved through closed reduction but will not maintain alignment, percutaneous fixation can be used to maintain correction. If anatomic reduction cannot be achieved by closed reduction, soft tissue interposition may be present and should be corrected before inserting fixation.

Metatarsal fractures have two different mechanisms of injury: direct trauma and indirect trauma. Direct trauma is caused by a crush injury or a sudden impact. Indirect trauma includes torque injuries, abnormal biomechanical forces, or traction forces [15]. Torque injuries usually occur when the leg and hindfoot are twisted with the forefoot in a fixed position [16].

The goal of reduction is to realign the anatomic relationship of the metatarsals. Some displacement of metatarsal fractures can be tolerated, especially in the frontal plane. Transverse plane displacement at the metatarsal head–neck level may cause mechanical impingement and neuroma formation. Sagittal plane displacement may alter the weight-bearing distribution of the metatarsal heads. Plantar displacement may add additional pressure, causing metatarsalgia or painful hyperkeratotic lesions. Dorsal displacement may

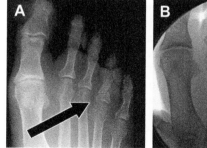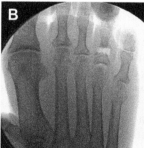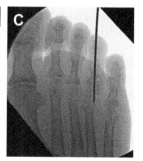

Fig. 1. (*A*) Anterior-posterior weight-bearing radiograph of a 68-year-old man who had uncontrolled diabetes, peripheral neuropathy, a long smoking history, and a 6-week history of fractured fourth proximal phalanx (*black arrow*). (*B*) Intraoperative image intensification view after a small curette was delivered through a percutaneous incision to remove sclerotic debris from the fracture site. (*C*) Allogenic bone matrix containing viable adult mesenchymal stem cells (Trinity Matrix; Blackstone Medical, Inc., Springfield, Massachusetts) was inserted into the debrided fracture site, followed by antegrade delivery of a small-diameter Kirschner wire across the metatarsophalangeal joint to stabilize the fracture fragment.

transfer pressure to adjacent metatarsal heads. Additionally, fractures of the first and fifth metatarsals may have additional consequences, such as hallux valgus and digitus quintus varus deformities [17].

Often, with highly comminuted metatarsal fractures, small fragments exist that are difficult to align and do not typically allow for screw purchase. Although open reduction internal fixation is the standard technique used to obtain anatomic alignment of metatarsal fractures, it often requires significant soft tissue exposure, which may lead to osseous devascularization and soft tissue necrosis in the high-risk patient. Although percutaneous wires do not provide active compression, they are more than adequate for stabilization purposes for most metatarsal fractures. When performing percutaneous pinning of metatarsal fractures, Kirschner wires should first be inserted into the unstable fragment and then into the stable fragment [18]. If performed in the reverse order, the Kirschner wire can push the unstable fragment away from the desired position. Care must be taken in the selection of Kirschner wire use because these wires do not resist rotational forces unless multiple wires are used at some obliquity [18] and because they do not resist bending forces, especially in transverse shaft fractures [19].

First metatarsal fractures

The first metatarsal is less commonly injured than other metatarsals because of its relative strength, size, and mobility. It bears greater forces than any other single metatarsal during ambulation. If anatomic alignment is lost, the function of the first metatarsal during propulsion can be compromised. Therefore, reduction of the fracture in all three cardinal planes is paramount, to maintain function. It is also important to realign all angular, rotational, and length deformities [16–19].

Although intramedullary pinning of the first metatarsal is effective with open fixation, several other techniques can be used in a purely percutaneous approach. Smooth or threaded Kirschner wires and percutaneous cannulated screws work well for first metatarsal head fractures. Crossed Kirschner wires or external fixation can be useful with severe comminution of the first metatarsal because open reduction does not allow for purchase of small fragments. Transmetatarsal wire fixation or external fixation can be useful for maintaining length and stability of the first metatarsal. These techniques are beneficial when metatarsal length is lost [16–19].

Central metatarsal fractures

Fractures of the second, third, or fourth metatarsals are inherently more stable than fractures of the first or fifth metatarsals because of the intrinsic muscular attachments and ligamentous structures supporting the metatarsals. Central metatarsal fractures are often seen in conjunction with other metatarsal and midtarsal injuries.

When central metatarsal neck fractures are displaced, traction can be placed on the metatarsals to bring them back to length. With subcapital fractures, the head tends to move plantarly, whereas in oblique fractures of the shaft, the head tends to shorten [16]. A technique that works particularly well for multiple metatarsal fractures is the concept of buttressing. A Kirschner wire is inserted into the distal lateral fifth metatarsal and advanced through the fractured metatarsal heads using intraoperative image intensification [20]. The metatarsal fracture or fractures will be stabilized using the intact fifth metatarsal as a buttress.

Retrograde percutaneous pinning is the gold standard surgical treatment of choice for noncomminuted fractures of the central metatarsals [17]. A Kirschner wire is inserted through the distal phalanx under image intensification and is advanced through the digit, into the metatarsal head, and then into the shaft. Rammelt and colleagues [16] recommend holding the head of the proximal phalanx with a sharp reduction clamp percutaneously for better control of the distal fragment and toe.

Proximal fifth metatarsal fractures

Proximal fifth metatarsal fractures occur in three distinct regions: the tuberosity (ie, avulsion), the base (ie, area of the fourth–fifth intermetatarsal articulation), and the metaphyseal-diaphyseal region (ie, Jones-type). Recent literature has reported higher patient satisfaction with surgical intervention for fifth metatarsal shaft fractures, avulsion fractures, and metaphyseal-diaphyseal fractures than with prolonged casting [21].

Tuberosity avulsion fractures (ie, tennis fractures) are the most common fifth metatarsal fracture [22]. The mechanism of injury typically results from ankle inversion while the foot is in plantar flexion. These patients may report a history of an ankle sprain. The pathogenesis of fractures of the proximal portion of the fifth metatarsal bone appears to be related to avulsion injury of the lateral component of the plantar aponeurosis and theperoneus brevis tendon fibers [23].

Avulsion fractures tend to heal with non–weight-bearing short leg cast immobilization. Dameron [24] found that fifth metatarsal avulsion fractures were clinically united within 3 weeks and radiographically united within 2 months, but the study does not describe long-term functional outcome. Patients treated nonsurgically make take 6 months or longer to return to their preinjury level of function, based on a study by Egol and colleagues [25], which reported that only 20% of the patients studied returned to preinjury functional status by 3 months and 86% by 6 months, and it took 1 year for all patients to reach preinjury status. Vorlat and colleagues [26] concluded that the most significant predictor of poor functional outcome in avulsion fractures was prolonged non–weight bearing, which was strongly associated with worse global outcome, discomfort, and stiffness. For these reasons, the investigators recommended that non–weight bearing be kept to a minimum for acute avulsions of the tuberosity of the fifth metatarsal.

They believed that internal fixation provided a construct that allowed for earlier weight bearing in these patients [26].

The authors' choice for fixation of avulsion fractures in the high-risk patient is a single percutaneous bicortical cancellous screw. This technique provides adequate rigid internal fixation with a decrease in the potential complications associated with open reduction internal fixation in the high-risk patient (Fig. 2). When this technique was compared with an open approach using tension band stabilization, the percutaneous screw fixation created increased stability across the fracture site [27,28].

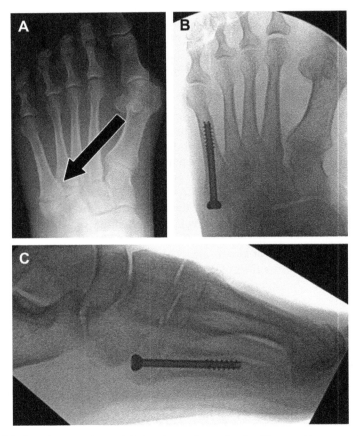

Fig. 2. (*A*) Anterior-posterior weight-bearing radiograph of a 63-year-old woman who had a history of insulin-dependent diabetes and longstanding tobacco abuse and a 5-week history of a fifth metatarsal avulsion fracture (*black arrow*). Using the technique described by Roukis and colleagues [28] to provide reduction of the fracture and delivery of internal fixation, a 4.0-mm partially threaded cancellous screw was percutaneously inserted for fixation of the fracture, as demonstrated on the anterior-posterior (*B*) and lateral (*C*) intraoperative image intensification views.

Transverse proximal diaphyseal (ie, Jones-type) fractures are extra-articular and are located approximately 1.5 to 3 cm distal to the tuberosity of the fifth metatarsal [29]. These fractures typically result from vertical or medial-lateral force on the fifth metatarsal base while the patient's weight is over the lateral aspect of the plantar-flexed foot [30]. Transverse proximal diaphyseal fractures are notorious for a variable and prolonged course of healing, clinically and radiographically [24]. Mologone and colleagues [31] reported a 44% failure after cast treatment of acute transverse proximal diaphyseal fractures [31]. Konkel and colleagues [32] reported an average of 3.5 months to osseous union and recommended nonoperative treatment of transverse proximal diaphyseal fractures for patients in which time to return to work was not critical.

Surgical fixation of transverse proximal diaphyseal fractures results in a quicker recovery time for radiographic union and a quicker return to normal activity, compared with cast immobilization [31]. With internal fixation, patients can return to full activity levels 6 to 8 weeks postopera-tively [30,31]. The percutaneous technique for fixation of a transverse prox-imal diaphyseal fracture is identical to the technique mentioned previously for fifth metatarsal tuberosity avulsion fractures. In one study, fixation with a stainless steel 4.5-mm cannulated screw provided 100% clinical healing and near 100% healing radiographically [33]. Although Arangio [34] has discussed a percutaneous crossed wire approach, the authors' preferred technique in the high-risk patient is percutaneous cannulated screw fixation.

Cuboid fracture-dislocations

Fracture-dislocations to the cuboid are rare, accounting for 5% of all midfoot fractures [35]. Typically, they occur with other midfoot fracture-dislocations but they can also be found as isolated injuries [36–41]. Fractures may result from direct injuries (ie, crush) or indirect injuries (ie, twisting and impaction) through traction across capsular and ligamentous attachments. Fractures are categorized as avulsion, body fracture-dislocations, and stress fractures [35]. The most common cuboid fracture, occurring 66% of the time, is a chip fracture or avulsion from the plantar calcaneocuboid liga-ment [35]. The classic cuboid injury is a "nutcracker fracture," as described by Hermel and Gershon-Cohen [42]. This compression fracture occurs when the forefoot is forcibly everted on the hindfoot and the cuboid is compressed between the base of the fourth and fifth metatarsals and the anterior calca-neus [42]. Associated injuries may include fracture of the navicular tuberos-ity or posterior tibial tendon tear [36,43]. Surgical treatment is of particular importance because the cuboid has a central role in maintaining the integrity of the lateral column. If cuboid fractures are left untreated, disabling post-traumatic arthritis and a painful flatfoot deformity caused by shortening of the lateral column can occur [37,44]. After healing of a cuboid fracture, peroneal longus tendon dysfunction has been reported, caused by scarring of the tendon and disruption of the peroneal groove [35,45].

Localized tenderness over the dorsal lateral foot, with significant swelling and a history of direct or indirect trauma to the midfoot, should raise the suspicion of a midfoot injury. Also, a painful and stiff subtalar joint range of motion with a freely movable ankle joint should raise the index of suspicion for a fracture [35]. Initial imaging includes anterier-posterior, lateral, and lateral-oblique radiographs. A 30° medial oblique view may be beneficial because it allows the cuboid and surrounding joints to be visualized without overlapping projections [46]. The lateral-oblique radiograph allows visualization of any pathology present, without overlap. If surgery is planned, a CT scan is beneficial to evaluate the fracture anatomy and surrounding midfoot joint involvement.

Maintaining length and mobility of the lateral column are two important keys to successful treatment of cuboid fractures [43]. Typically, compression fractures with articular incongruity and displacement are treated with open reduction and internal fixation, with insertion of a structural bone graft [38,47]. In a high-risk patient who may not tolerate an open procedure with extensive soft tissue dissection, percutaneous options are available, although published literature is not available on the outcomes and healing of percutaneous internal fixation of cuboid fractures. Dislocations of the cuboid have been treated successfully with percutaneous reduction and fixation [41]. Most reported dislocations underwent open reduction with percutaneous fixation because of entrapment of surrounding tendons [36–41,43]. Stress fractures and nondisplaced fractures do well with 4 to 6 weeks of cast immobilization [48,49], but compression and displaced fractures are doomed to failure and disability with immobilization alone [38].

Total dislocations have been treated successfully with closed reduction and percutaneous fixation with Kirschner wires [41]. The cuboid is reduced by inverting the foot to open the space that normally occupies the cuboid, and manual pressure can be applied to the body of the cuboid to aid in reduction. Also, a small stab incision can be placed and a periosteal elevator can be used to "toggle" the cuboid into the space that it normally occupies [43]. A 4.0-mm cancellous screw can also be placed in the body of the cuboid to lever it back into place. The foot is then everted and lateral pressure is applied until Kirschner wires are inserted. Percutaneous Kirschner wires are driven across the body of the cuboid and into the calcaneus and lateral cuneiform for extraosseous stability. Non–weight bearing is maintained for 6 weeks and the Kirschner wires are removed [41].

For displaced fractures of the cuboid, an external fixator can be used to aid in indirect reduction of the articular incongruity. Estaugh-Waring and Saleh [50] described in a case report a technique for indirect reduction of a severely displaced cuboid fracture with a circular frame external fixator. The main importance of using the fixator was to restore the length of the lateral column through distraction while maintaining the integrity of the skin. Percutaneous Kirschner wires can then be used to stabilize the larger fracture fragments to the metatarsal bases or lateral cuneiform.

Tarsal-metatarsal joint fracture-dislocations

Injuries to the tarsal-metatarsal joint (ie, Lisfranc) are uncommon. The incidence is 0.2% to 0.9% of all fractures and occurs in 1 person per 55,000 each year [51–54]. Most of these injuries occur in patients polytraumatized by motor vehicle accidents, followed by those with crushing injuries and falls from heights [55,56]. Reports of missed tarsal-metatarsal joint injuries range from 20% to 30% [55,56].

The anatomy of the tarsal-metatarsal joint has been well described [52,57,58]. The articulations of the cuneiforms and metatarsals are trapezoidal in shape and form an arch to prevent dorsal dislocation. The second metatarsal is the keystone of the metatarsal arch and is recessed between the medial and lateral cuneiforms to provide additional stability. The key to reduction of a fracture-dislocation is the second metatarsal. In addition to the osseous stability, ligaments surrounding the tarsal-metatarsal joint provide stability. The lesser metatarsals are bound by the intermetatarsal ligaments. The Lisfranc ligament attaches the second metatarsal to the medial cuneiform. The dorsal and the stronger plantar transverse ligaments enhance stability and reduce the possibility of a dislocation.

Several classifications have been used to describe tarsal-metatarsal joint injuries [55,59,60]. No classification is considered the "standard" or tends to help more with preoperative planning. The mechanism of injury is either indirect or direct, with indirect injuries being more common [54].

Severely displaced fractures are easily diagnosed. They usually present with plantar ecchymosis at the midfoot level and the inability to bear weight on the affected foot [61]. More subtle injuries may not have obvious displacement or ecchymosis but will have tenderness along the medial midfoot. Also, stressing the tarsal-metatarsal joint by passively abducting and pronating the forefoot while keeping the hindfoot fixed with the opposite hand will elicit pain across the tarsal-metatarsal joint injury [62]. In any fracture-dislocation, assessing neurovascular status is important. The dorsalis pedis artery and deep peroneal nerve can be compromised and can cause hemorrhage or compartment syndrome [52,63], especially with crushing injuries where measurement of forefoot compartments may be indicated [52].

The initial radiographic analysis includes anterior-posterior, lateral-oblique, and lateral foot views. Normal and abnormal radiographic analyses have been clearly described in the literature (see Refs. [35,43,52,55,57,58]). The most common radiographic finding after a tarsal-metatarsal joint injury is diastasis (≥2 mm) between the bases of the first and second metatarsals. A pathognomonic finding is a "fleck" sign, which is seen in the space between the first and second metatarsals and represents avulsion of Lisfranc ligament. This finding has been reported in 90% of cases [55].

In more subtle injuries, contralateral weight-bearing comparison views can be helpful in evaluating any diastasis between the bases of the first and second metatarsals. In a highly suspicious injury where plain films are negative, a CT scan or MRI may show occult fractures or injuries to the Lisfranc ligament [64]. CT scanning can help determine fracture patterns and identify subtle malalignments and other associated midfoot fractures [65]. Stress views of the affected foot can be obtained [66]. In rare instances in which plain films are negative and advanced imaging is equivocal, stress views can be obtained under sedation in the operating room setting using image intensification to determine the laxity of the tarsal-metatarsal joint complex. This technique is done by pronating and forcibly abducting the forefoot with one hand and keeping the hindfoot fixed with the opposite hand then adducting/supinating the forefoot. If diastasis occurs between the first and second metatarsals, percutaneous fixation can be placed.

Anatomic reduction and stable fixation have become the standard for tarsal-metatarsal joint fracture-dislocations, to limit posttraumatic arthritis [35,43,52,53,58]. Most have agreed that stable anatomic reduction leads to optimal results [53,55,58,67]. Treatment with cast immobilization alone has generally resulted in poor results, such as extended immobilization, loss of reduction, and eventual need for arthrodesis [54–56,59,68]. Some investigators feel that nonoperative treatment does not have a role for any patient who has a tarsal-metatarsal joint injury [55,56].

Operative treatment of tarsal-metatarsal joint fracture-dislocations has evolved over the years. Fixation techniques vary throughout the literature. Historically, closed reduction without fixation resulted in poor results [54,56,59,68]. Closed reduction with percutaneous pin/screw fixation or open reduction and internal fixation are currently recommended over cast immobilization [55,56,58,59]. A recent cadaveric biomechanical study measured stiffness and displacement of three types of fixation placed across the tarsal-metatarsal joint complex [69]. The groups included four Kirschner wires, three cortical screws plus two Kirschner wires laterally, or five cortical screws. The investigator concluded that three cortical screws for the medial tarsal-metatarsal joints plus two Kirschner wires for the lateral tarsal-metatarsal joints resulted in greater stiffness than four Kirschner wires [69]. Pin tract infections, migration, and loss of reduction are all causes of unsuccessful reduction after using Kirschner wires [35]. Dorsal plating has also been described to treat displaced tarsal-metatarsal joint injuries and represents an alternative to transarticular screw placement [70]. However, the need for extensive soft tissue dissection and possible shoe wear irritation are disadvantages of bulky plating for tarsal-metatarsal joint injuries. Currently, open reduction to remove bone fragments, interposed capsule, or cartilage and to confirm the accuracy of reduction with direct exposure is advocated (See Refs. [43,53,55,67,70,71]). Once open reduction is obtained, rigid transarticular fixation is recommended to maintain the reduction [51–53,67,70]. Transarticular screws can be placed percutaneously. In a high-risk patient, surgical management with closed reduction and percutaneous fixation may be the most appropriate option to limit devitalization of the soft tissue envelope. Long-term results of patients undergoing percutaneous internal fixation of tarsal-metatarsal fracture-dislocations are available but do not include information specific to the high-risk patient.

Percutaneous reduction is first attained through longitudinal traction achieved by placing the toes in finger traps and applying traction at the ankle joint. Transverse and sagittal plane correction is then reduced manually with digital pressure. Also dorsiflexing the toes at the metatarsophalangeal joints creates stability at the tarsal-metatarsal joint by engaging the plantar fascia and flexor tendons [58]. Once the fracture is anatomically reduced, a large periarticular reduction forceps is placed percutaneously between the medial cuneiform and the base of the second metatarsal to stabilize the articulation (Fig. 3). Intraoperative image intensification is used to verify anatomic reduction, which consists of less than or equal to 2 mm of space between the first and second metatarsal, no lateral shifting of the third, fourth, and fifth metatarsals, and less than a 15° angle at the lateral tarsal-metatarsal axis [55,57]. The most important part of this procedure is to stabilize and reduce the second metatarsal into its recess.

The authors' preferred approach is to place rigid fixation in the medial three tarsal-metatarsal joints and the intercuneiform joints. Typically, small fragment, partially threaded, cannulated screws are used to achieve rigid fixation. First, the cuneiform instability typically associated with

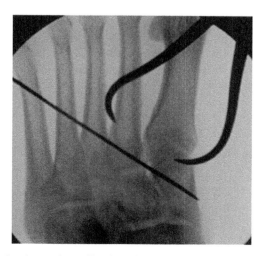

Fig. 3. Intraoperative image intensification view following closed reduction of a tarsal-metatarsal joint fracture-dislocation and application of a large periarticular reduction forceps percutaneously placed between the medial cuneiform and the base of the second metatarsal.

tarsal-metatarsal joint injury is stabilized by advancing a guidewire from the central-medial aspect of the medial cuneiform across the intercuneiform articulations and into the lateral cuneiform. A percutaneous incision is made at the wire insertion site, blunt dissection is carried to bone, and the small fragment screw is placed. Next, another guidewire is driven from the proximal-medial aspect of the medial cuneiform to the distal-lateral aspect of the second metatarsal, referred to as the "Lisfranc screw." The authors prefer this screw placement in a lag fashion to recreate the normal stabilizing effect of the Lisfranc ligament. A separate percutaneous incision is made at the wire, blunt dissection is carried to bone, and the small fragment screw is placed. The first tarsal-metatarsal joint is fixated next by driving a guidewire, starting in the dorsal-central first metatarsal and into the plantar-medial cuneiform. The third tarsal-metatarsal articulation is fixated by driving a guidewire from the dorsal-lateral aspect of the third metatarsal base into the lateral cuneiform in a dorsal-to-plantar direction. If needed, the fourth and fifth tarsal-metatarsal joints are fixated with two smooth Kirschner wires. Next, the large periarticular reduction forceps is removed and the reduction and stability are assessed using image intensification. The percutaneous incisions are typically closed with 4-0 nylon in a simple interrupted suture technique. A bulky, well-padded dressing is placed with a plaster sugar tong splint. This percutaneous technique allows anatomic reduction and placement of rigid internal fixation without disruption of the soft tissue envelope and with minimal complications (Fig. 4). Cast immobilization is maintained for 4 to 6 weeks to allow adequate osseous and ligamentous healing, at which time any Kirschner wires are removed in the office under aseptic technique. Once the cast is removed, patients are placed into a short leg walking cast for an additional 3 to 4 weeks. After this time, physical therapy is initiated and accommodative in-shoe orthoses are fabricated for shock absorption. Patients are typically fully weight bearing in a stiff shoe with the accommodative in-shoe orthoses by 12 weeks postoperatively. The screws are usually removed 4 to 12 months postoperatively to prevent screw breakage and further cartilage damage. However, in the high-risk patient, a second surgery may not be indicated to retrieve the fixation, to avoid iatrogenic injury.

Cuneiform fracture-dislocations

Cuneiform fractures most commonly occur in conjunction with other midfoot injuries [35,43]. Isolated cuneiform fracture-dislocations are rare, although they have been reported and account for 4.3% of all tarsal bone fractures [43,71,72]. Dislocations of the cuneiforms are rare, in part, because of the stability of stout ligaments and surrounding tendons such as the posterior tibial, anterior tibial, and peroneus longus tendons [35]. Dislocations have been reported, with associated injuries to the tarsal-metatarsal and midtarsal (ie, Chopart) joints [73]. The medial cuneiform appears to be

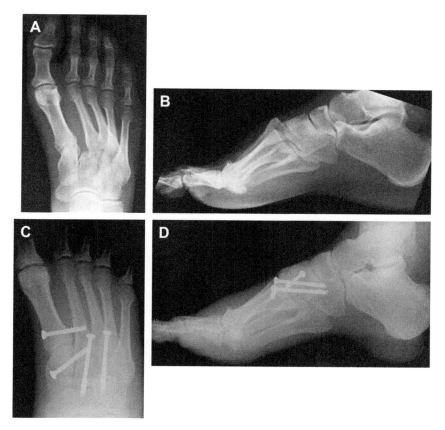

Fig. 4. Non–weight-bearing anterior-posterior (*A*) and lateral (*B*) radiographs of a 40-year-old uncontrolled diabetic man with a 20-year history of tobacco abuse, who sustained a tarsal-metatarsal fracture-dislocation in a motor vehicle accident. Partial weight-bearing postoperative anterior-posterior (*C*) and lateral (*D*) radiographs following delivery of percutaneous internal fixation consisting of multiple 4.0-mm cannulated partially threaded screws.

the most commonly injured of the three cuneiforms [43]. A fracture can be categorized as a chip fracture, caused by avulsion of the anterior tibial tendon, or a crush fracture, caused by a direct injury [71]. A tarsal-metatarsal joint variant can occur with a medial cuneiform fracture-dislocation when the intercuneiform joint and first metatarsal interspace are injured [43]. Standard radiographs and CT scan should be obtained preoperatively to assess the location and extent of injury.

Typically, displaced cuneiform fractures are treated with open reduction and lag screw fixation [35,43]. Reduction can be difficult at times because of an entrapped tibialis anterior tendon [74]. In a high-risk patient, percutaneous reduction and fixation may be the most appropriate alternative; however, only a few cases have been reported [75]. After reduction, fractures and dislocations can be stabilized with percutaneous Kirschner wires, Stein-mann pins, or cannulated lag screws [43,76]. Pinney and Sangeorzan [43,76] suggests that fixation can be driven across intercuneiform joints and into surrounding metatarsal bases for stabilization. Cannulated lag screws are placed from medial to lateral and advanced into the surrounding cuneiforms or metatarsal bases. Long-term fixation is needed for stability because of the extensive ligament damage [43]. If a rare intermediate cuneiform dislocation is encountered, it is essential to reduce the fracture-dislocation anatomically because it serves as the keystone to the transverse arch [43]. Mini external fixation or temporary distraction can be used to span fractures and stabilize dislocations, after which percutaneous internal fixation can be placed. Patients are placed in a non–weight-bearing short leg cast for 6 to 8 weeks. Percutaneous Kirschner wires are removed 6 weeks postoperatively in the office under aseptic technique.

Navicular fracture-dislocations

The navicular plays a major role in stabilizing the medial longitudinal arch and navicular fracture-dislocations carry high morbidity if not diag-nosed and treated appropriately. Navicular fractures can vary in severity from isolated dislocations and avulsion fractures to comminuted fracture-dislocations of the body. Displaced fractures are rare because of the surrounding plantar and dorsal ligaments [77]. Isolated dislocations of the navicular are a rare phenomenon, especially if no fracture is associated with the dislocation [78]. Although a rare injury, navicular dislocations occur with high-energy trauma, such as a motor vehicle accident, and in combination with other tarsal dislocations [78]. A navicular fracture can be classified inherently as a "high-risk" fracture because of its blood supply. Torg and colleagues [79] described the navicular blood supply and deter-mined that it is well vascularized at the periphery but avascular centrally. Vessels that supply the navicular originate from the dorsalis pedis and medial plantar artery and enter through the tuberosity.

Accessory ossicles such as os supratalare and os tibiale externum must be distinguished from a fracture. Os tibiale externum is present in 15% to 25% of the population and is bilateral 90% of the time [80]. A synchondritic joint ties the accessory ossicle to the navicular and this joint can fracture in adults, causing medial arch pain and edema that can mimic a fracture [80].

Several types of navicular fractures exist [79,81]. The most common, oc-curring 47% of the time, is an avulsion fracture of the dorsal lip, according to Eichenholtz and Levine [81]. The avulsion fracture occurs because of a plantar flexion force that creates tension of the dorsal talar-navicular ligament or deltoid ligament [80,81]. For nondisplaced fractures, treatment usually consists of immobilization in a short leg cast for 4 to 6 weeks. Exci-sion can be considered in displaced, small, and symptomatic avulsion fractures. Percutaneous Kirschner wire fixation has been described for those fractures that are greater than or equal to one quarter of the articular surface, to restore the talar-navicular joint congruity [35].

Tuberosity fractures account for 2% to 12% of navicular fractures [82]. The posterior tibial tendon and fibers of the deltoid ligament can cause tuberosity fractures with forced eversion of the foot [35]. Associated injuries, such as a cuboid, calcaneal anterior process fracture or subluxation of the midtarsal joint, can occur in conjunction with a navicular tuberosity fracture [81]. Typically, tuberosity fractures are nondisplaced because of multiple ligament attachments and the broad posterior tibial tendon insertion [82]. Bone scintigraphy or MRI can be helpful in the diagnosis of a symptomatic accessory ossicle without a history of trauma. An accessory ossicle usually does not require surgical intervention, but a displaced tuberosity fracture does, to prevent a late dorsal-lateral peritalar subluxation (ie, collapsed pes plano valgus) deformity. A percutaneous guidewire can be placed in the displaced tuberosity fragment and used as a "toggle" to mobilize and reduce the fracture. Once reduced, the pin can be driven further into the navicular for fixation and a second pin can be added for fracture stability. Alternatively, two small cannulated screws can be placed for rigid internal fixation. Patients are maintained in a non–weight-bearing cast for 6 weeks. In-shoe orthoses may be beneficial postoperatively to support the medial longitudinal arch.

Body fractures are the most infrequent navicular fracture. Fractures that occur from a direct force are isolated and comminuted but usually not displaced [35]. Indirect forces such as a motor vehicle accident or a fall from a height on a plantar-flexed foot result in displaced fractures. Multiple radiographs and a CT scan must be obtained to determine fracture patterns and degree of comminution.

Sangeorzan and colleagues [77] classified body fractures into three types, based on position and displacement of fragments and foot. Type 1 and 2 fractures can have one fracture line; however, the foot is medially deviated in type 2 fractures. A comminuted fracture with disruption of the medial column and a laterally deviated forefoot exists in a type 3 fracture. Treatment goals in all three types of fractures are to restore the medial column and preserve the talar-navicular joint alignment. Open reduction and internal fixation through an anterior-medial approach is recommend for all three types of fractures. Navicular body fractures are inherently high risk because of lack of blood supply within the central portion and, according to Sangeorzan and colleagues [77], avascular necrosis occurs in 25% of these fractures. Excessive soft tissue stripping and further devascularization can be avoided with percutaneous internal fixation. In a high-risk patient, percutaneous internal fixation may represent the only viable option. No published peer-reviewed literature is available regarding percutaneous internal fixation in a high-risk patient.

In type 1 fractures, dorsal and plantar fracture fragments occur in the coronal plane through the body of the navicular. Provisional reduction and fixation can be achieved through percutaneous threaded pins or Kirschner wires. If needed, a small incision can be created over the central navicular to insert an elevator to mobilize and reduce the fracture fragment. Rigid internal fixation using small cannulated lag screws are placed from superior to inferior through the body. The provisional fixation is removed and the patient is placed in a non–weight-bearing cast for 6 weeks.

In type 2 fractures, the major fracture line extends from dorsal-lateral to plantar-medial through the navicular. The medial column has shortened and the forefoot is displaced medially. According to Sangeorzan and colleagues [77], the length of the medial column must be restored to reduce the fracture accurately. Distraction and reduction of the medial column can be achieved by placing a mini external fixator from the talus to the base of the first metatarsal. Provisional fixation and reduction of the talonavicular joint alignment can be achieved through Kirschner wires or pins. Percutaneous cannulated lag screws are driven from the large medial fragment into the lateral navicular. At times, comminution at the plantar-lateral aspect of the navicular makes this screw position difficult. Instead, the medial fragment can be fixated to the adjacent cuneiforms [35,80]. The mini external fixator is left in place as adjunct fixation and to distract the medial column during fracture healing. Transarticular fixation and the mini external fixator are removed after union is accomplished before initiating weight bearing and mobilization, which are begun approximately 8 weeks postoperatively.

Type 3 fractures involve comminution of the navicular body with disruption of the medial column, and the forefoot is laterally displaced. Fixation is much like that used for type 2 fractures, with the use of a mini external fixator to restore the medial column and assist in fracture reduction. Multiple Kirschner wires for transfixation of the navicular-cuneiform and talonavicular joints are required [35]. Fixation devices are removed at 8 weeks before initiating mobilization. Postoperatively, patients are non–weight bearing until clinical and radiographic union is achieved.

According to Romash [80], custom in-shoe orthoses are dispensed postoperatively with 70% good results [80]. An electric bone growth stimulator (Combined Magnetic Field Bone Growth Stimulation, OL 1000 SC Size 3; DONJOY Orthopaedics, LLC, Vista, California) can be used until consolidation of the fracture is noted.

Calcaneal fractures

Calcaneal fractures are the most common of the tarsal bone fractures [4,83]. Extra-articular fractures are encountered approximately 75% of the time and can usually be treated conservatively [6]. The remaining 25% are intra-articular in nature and require surgical management as the definitive treatment [6]. These intra-articular fractures are the result of a high-velocity injury, such as a fall from a height [9]. The potential complications of subtalar arthritis, chronic pain, and peroneal tendonitis seen with intra-articular calcaneal fractures are increased with nonoperative treatment [6,10]. These poor results with nonoperative methods created a shift to operative management for these injuries.

Intra-articular calcaneal fractures are most commonly treated by open reduction internal fixation though an extensile lateral incision [4]. The characteristics of an intra-articular calcaneal fracture increase the potential risks associated with open reduction internal fixation [10]. The most common complications are dehiscence and infection, which are byproducts of the limited soft tissue envelope surrounding the calcaneus and the extensive soft tissue damage associated with the high-velocity nature of these injuries [7,10]. In high-risk patients, these potential complications are increased. Minimum incision or percutaneous fixation techniques for intra-articular fractures of the calcaneus represent viable surgical options for these high-risk patients [7,10].

Two fracture patterns for intra-articular calcaneal fractures have been described: tongue type and joint depression. The tongue-type fracture maintains the continuity between the posterior facet and the calcaneal tuberosity. Joint depression fractures involve a separation of the posterior facet from the tuberosity. Because of the large fragment noted with the tongue-type fracture, reduction of this segment will indirectly reduce the posterior facet and restore Böhler's angle. For this reason, the tongue-type fracture is more amenable to percutaneous fixation methods [4,7,10].

The percutaneous fixation techniques for calcaneal fractures can be divided into two categories: traction and pin leverage/screw fixation [7]. Both techniques involve indirect reduction and subsequent percutaneous stabilization with the assistance of intra-operative image intensification. Traction involves the concept of "ligamentotaxis" to reduce the fracture, which is achieved with the use of a pin introduced through the posterior tuberosity of the calcaneus from medial to lateral to provide skeletal traction, or with the use of a spanning external fixator to provide skeletal traction, which aids fracture alignment and reduction [7]. Specifically, the pin is used to provide manual traction to reduce the varus deformity of the heel and to provide length and decrease width of the calcaneus. Intra-operative image intensification is used to obtain calcaneal-axial and Bröden views to assess reduction. If adequate reduction of the posterior facet is not obtained, an elevator is subsequently inserted percutaneously to raise the depressed posterior facet, followed by application of a large periarticular reduction forceps to reduce the width of the calcaneus. If adequate reduction of the tuberosity fragment is still not obtained, pin leverage/screw fixation is used, which involves insertion of a reduction pin into the main portion of the tuberosity fragment in line with the superior border of the calcaneus, to reduce the fragment. Intraoperative image intensification is used to verify proper reduction, followed by insertion of provisional fixation with the use of percutaneously inserted Kirschner wires or cannulated guidewires [7,84,85]. Permanent fixation is then achieved with the use of cannulated lag screws of between 4.0 and 7.3 mm, depending on the size and number of fracture fragments, inserted lateral to medial from the lateral cortical wall to the sustentaculum tali or medial cortical wall, with care taken not to violate the medial neurovascular and tendinous structures. The authors advocate either method of percutaneous fixation for reduction and stabilization of calcaneal fractures in the high-risk patient (Fig. 5).

With tongue-type fractures, fixation is inserted from the plantar tuberosity into the tongue fragment to counteract the upward traction of the Achilles tendon [7,10]. Percutaneous fixation in each method is aimed at reduction of the fracture fragments to the inherently stable superior-medial sustentaculum tali fragment [10].

Multiple literature entries review percutaneous fixation techniques for intra-articular calcaneal fractures [4,7,10]. Although some of these reports mention the high-risk patient who has an intra-articular calcaneal fracture as an indication for percutaneous fixation [4,7,10], none specifically differentiate their results in the high-risk patient population. In 1998, Tornetta [84] reported the results of 22 patients who had a tongue-type fracture (ie, Sanders type II-C) treated with percutaneous leverage based on the Essex-Lopresti reduction technique. The patients were followed for an average of 2.9 years, with good to excellent results in 87% of the patients, according to the Maryland Foot Score. Pin tract infections were reported in 4 of 17 (24%) patients, prompting a change in fixation from Steinman pins to cannulated screws. In 2000, Tornetta [85] further reported good to excellent results in 41 patients who had Sanders type II-C fractures, using the same method. He concluded that Sanders type II-C fractures are best suited for percutaneous fixation [85].

Stulik and colleagues [10] described their method of minimally invasive treatment of intra-articular calcaneal fractures in 2006. They reported the results of 287 intra-articular fractures of the calcaneus in 247 patients. These fractures included 175 Sanders type II fractures, 86 Sanders type III fractures, and 26 Sanders type IV fractures, and 183 joint depression fractures, 72 tongue-type fractures, and 32 comminuted fractures. The fractures were treated using a standard protocol of semi-open reduction and Kirschner wire fixation. A 4.5-mm Steinmann pin was inserted into the posterior-inferior portion of the calcaneal tuberosity and skeletal traction was applied to lengthen the calcaneus and reduce the varus deformity of the heel. With a joint depression fracture, a stab incision was made in the sole of the foot and the posterior facet was elevated and reduced. In a tongue-type fracture, a 3- to 4-mm Steinmann pin was inserted lateral to the Achilles tendon and used to lever the posterior facet into alignment. With reduction confirmed, based on intra-operative image intensification, the fracture was held in place with two 2-mm Kirschner wires. The heel was then compressed and Kirschner wires inserted transversely from lateral to medial to the stable sustentaculum tali fragment. Finally, the overall reduction was obtained with six to eight 2-mm Kirschner wires that were cut flush to the skin. Pin tract infections were reported in 20 (7%) cases and deep infection with osteomyelitis in 5 (1.7%) cases. With the use of the Creighton-Nebraska Foundation score, 16.5% of the patients had an excellent result, 55.7% had good, 14.8% fair, and 13% poor. The results were slightly better with tongue-type fractures, with a median score of 86.5 out of 100, compared with joint depression fractures, with a median score of 81.2. The investigators offered four conclusions, based on their data and a review of the literature: (1) joint depression fractures are difficult to reduce; (2) tongue-type fractures can be treated successfully with minimally invasive techniques; (3) all Sanders type IV fractures should be treated with minimally invasive techniques; and (4) all displaced intra-articular fractures in high-risk patients can be treated safely with minimally invasive techniques [10].

In 2007, Schepers and colleagues [9] retrospectively reviewed 50 patients who had 61 intra-articular calcaneal fractures treated percutaneously. Each patient was placed in the prone position, with two intraoperative image intensification devices used. Three 3-mm Kirschner wires were placed lateral to medial through the calcaneal tuberosity, the cuboid, and the talar neck. A medial and lateral distractor was applied to the Kirschner wires. The Böhler's angle was restored with the use of these distractors and reduction was confirmed with intra-operative image intensification. If necessary, a blunt instrument was inserted into the plantar aspect of the foot to elevate any depressed segments of the subtalar joint surface of the calcaneus. Once adequate reduction was noted, two Kirschner wires or two cancellous screws were inserted from the posterior aspect of the tuberosity. The width of the calcaneus was then reduced with the addition of a third screw inserted from lateral into the sustentaculum tali. Seven (11.5%) patients had superficial wound infections, 2 (3%) patients developed deep infections, 1 (1.6%) developed a deep pin infection, and 1 (1.6%) developed osteomyelitis. The Maryland Foot Score indicated 28% excellent results, 32% good, 24% fair, and 16% poor. The Creighton-Nebraska Foundation score showed 18% excellent results, 24% good, 28% fair, and 30% poor. It was the investigators' conclusion that, because of the similar infection results of percutaneous fixation in comparison to open procedures, open procedures offer little benefit [9].

Talar fractures

Talar fractures are unique but uncommon fractures encountered by the foot and ankle surgeon. The distinct characteristics of the talus create a significant challenge for fracture management [86,87]. The anatomic location and the tenuous blood supply to the talus are major factors in the high rate of complications seen with a talar fracture [86,87]. The talus articulates with three joints: the ankle, subtalar, and talonavicular joints. Therefore, most of the talus is articular surface. These important anatomic characteristics necessitate meticulous surgical planning and management and exact

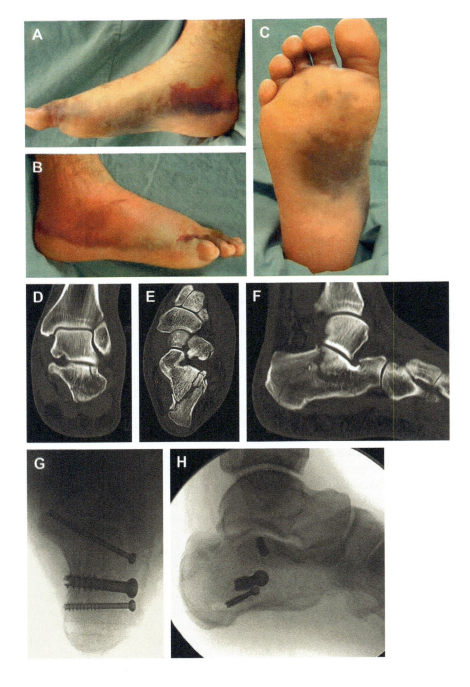

anatomic reconstruction, to decrease the possibility of posttraumatic complications [88]. This tenant of surgical management of the talus is more appropriately addressed through open reduction internal fixation. Open reduction internal fixation provides access and direct visualization of the fracture, thus assuring articular congruity and decreasing talar malalignment [88]. With an inability to visualize the talus directly and provide exact anatomic alignment with use of percutaneous fixation techniques, few references for percutaneous fixation for talar fractures are found in the literature. In the high-risk patient who has a talar fracture, the inability to provide adequate anatomic alignment with percutaneous fixation negates the advantages seen with percutaneous fixation for other fractures.

Although percutaneous fixation as an isolated surgical management for talar fractures is not advocated, the use of percutaneous fixation as an adjunct to open reduction of talar neck fractures is widely accepted. The classic open approach to reduction of the talar neck fracture is through an anterior-medial incision located between the anterior tibial and the extensor hallucis longus tendons. The fracture site is identified through this incision and the talus reduced under direct visualization. Temporary fixation is achieved through percutaneous Kirschner wire placement, after which the foot and leg are internally rotated and an anterior-lateral or posterior-lateral approach is used for placement of percutaneous fixation. When using the posterior-lateral approach, the entry point is identified posterior and parallel to the peroneal tendons. Using intra-operative image intensification, two cannulated guidewires are inserted slightly superior to the posterior talar process. The guidewires are driven from posterior to anterior into the talar head, perpendicular to the fracture site. Two 4.0- or 4.5-mm cannulated screws are inserted over the guidewires for permanent fixation. Sharma and colleagues [89] advocated the use of an anterior cruciate ligament tibial jig because of the challenging nature of the posterior-to-anterior approach for screw placement for talar neck fractures. These investigators indicated that the use of the jig would allow for insertion of internal fixation at desirable angles between 30° and 70° and would improve the accuracy of guidewire placement. Some concerns are associated with the use of this approach [86,87]. Deep dissection is required and injury to the posterior-lateral ankle structures may be encountered. A prominent screw head may impinge on the either the calcaneus or tibia with range of motion. With the anterior-lateral approach, either one cannulated guidewire is inserted anterior-lateral

Fig. 5. Medial (A), lateral (B), and plantar (C) clinical photographs of a 30-year-old male patient who had insulin-dependent diabetes and a 5-year history of tobacco abuse, who sustained a displaced intra-articular calcaneal fracture after falling down a flight of stairs. Preoperative frontal (D), transverse (E), and sagittal (F) CT images demonstrate the nature of the fracture. Intraoperative axial (G) and lateral (H) image intensification views following percutaneous fixation of the calcaneus with the use of one 7.3-mm cannulated screw and two 4.0-mm cannulated screws demonstrate the alignment and reduction achieved.

over the talar head along with one guidewire inserted through the anterior-medial incision, or both guidewires are inserted through the anterior-medial approach. Using intraoperative image intensification, two cannulated screw guidewires are inserted and driven from anterior to posterior into the talar head, perpendicular to the fracture site. Two 4.0- or 4.5-mm cannulated screws are inserted over the guidewires for permanent fixation. Titanium screws are recommended in talar fractures to allow improved image quality when using MRI postoperatively to monitor for avascular necrosis [87].

Ankle fractures

Ankle fractures in the high-risk patient, especially patients who have diabetes mellitus, have a history of being a clinical dilemma [76]. Issues with wound healing and fracture healing and the possibility of the development of Charcot neuro-osteoarthropathy in patients who have dense peripheral neuropathy create difficulty in determining the appropriate treatment protocol in high-risk patients. References in the literature regarding treatment protocols for ankle fractures in high-risk patients are scarce.

In 2001, Bibbo [90] provided an overview of complications from ankle fractures in diabetic patients. He reviewed available clinical series of diabetic ankle fractures treated with open reduction internal fixation. He provided three conclusions from a review of these clinical series: (1) diabetic fractures heal but significant delays in bone healing exist; (2) diabetic patients who have ankle fractures are at a high risk for wound complications; and (3) Charcot neuro-osteoarthropathy is more prevalent in patients misdiagnosed or treated late and in patients treated nonoperatively. From these conclusions, several clinical questions were presented and answered. A review of these answers can be adapted for the high-risk patient and as indications for percutaneous surgical management. Steps that can be taken to decrease the potential complications seen with open operative management of ankle fractures in the high-risk patient are early closed reduction of the fracture and delaying surgical reconstruction for a minimum of 10 days to allow for optimal medical management and viability of the soft tissue envelope.

The number of references in the literature regarding percutaneous fixation for ankle fractures is limited. In 1976, Hoffer [91] described his percutaneous technique for unstable ankle fractures. He advocated the concept of lateral malleolar transtibial pin fixation after reporting his results in 12 patients. Initially, any associated medial or posterior injury was repaired through a medial incision. A percutaneous smooth Steinmann pin was then inserted obliquely from the lateral malleolus into the tibia to stabilize the reduction. The pin was removed at 6 weeks and weight bearing was permitted. It was reported that all patients had good results and minimal pain and were able to return to work in 3 to 6 months [91].

A detailed analysis describing the use of percutaneous fixation of ankle fractures was reported by Ray and colleagues [8] in 1994. They retrospectively reviewed 24 patients who had Weber B and low Weber C ankle fractures treated with closed reduction and percutaneous internal fixation using an intramedullary, fully threaded, self-tapping screw. The investigators' rationale for the use of this percutaneous technique focused on complications secondary to the use of a lateral fibular plate, which included scarring, periosteal stripping, wound breakdown and infection secondary to the small soft tissue envelope of the lateral distal fibula. They also believed that articular cartilage damage or damage to the peroneal tendons were possibilities with the use of a lag screw and distal fibular plate. Indications for the procedure were a transverse or short oblique fracture of the lateral malleolus without any significant comminution noted. One nonunion and one superficial infection were encountered. Functional results were 42% excellent, 42% good, 5.3 % fair, and 10.5% poor.

Percutaneous reduction of ankle fractures is performed by internally rotating the foot to provide reduction, which is confirmed by way of intraoperative image intensification, followed by the placement of a large periarticular reduction forceps applied percutaneously to maintain reduction and provide stability. Once the fracture is reduced and stabilized, a percutaneous incision is made over the distal tip of the lateral malleolus and an entry hole in the distal fibula is made with a drill bit. A 4.0- or 4.5-mm cannulated self-tapping screw is placed across the fracture site and tightened until compression is achieved across the fracture site.

In 1999, Kim and Oh [92] reported their results with fixation of Danis-Weber type B fractures of the ankle using only one or two lag screws with minimal soft tissue dissection. Through this minimal incision, the lateral malleolus fracture was reduced and anatomically fixated with one or two 3.5-mm cortical lags screws. The investigators' main reason for using this technique was to decrease the potential for articular cartilage damage during the process of fixating a lateral plate to the distal fibula with screws. A non–weight-bearing below-the-knee cast was applied for an average of 4 weeks postoperatively, followed by full weight bearing at the fourth postoperative week. In 67 of 70 (96%) cases, the investigators were able to obtain anatomic reduction and stable fixation [92].

The authors' preferred method for fixation of ankle fractures in the high-risk patient is determined by the variables presented on a case-by-case basis, considering the fracture pattern, degree of soft tissue envelope injury, and quality of the bone before determining the method of treatment. Several accepted fixation methods for ankle fractures can be incorporated into percutaneous fixation for use in the high-risk patient. Cannulated screw fixation for medial malleolar fractures and distal tibial-fibular syndesmosis disruption, and intramedullary cannulated screw fixation for transverse or short oblique lateral malleolus fractures, may be used in the high-risk patient for osseous stabilization without compromising the fragile soft tissue envelope.

Tibial pilon fractures

Tibial pilon (ie, distal tibial plafond) fractures are a devastating injury to the lower extremity. The injury is the result of high-velocity trauma secondary to the talus impacting on the distal articular surface of the tibia [11]. The tibial pilon fracture is an intra-articular injury that occurs in 7% of tibial fractures [11]. As with fractures of the calcaneus, the high-impact nature of this injury severely compromises the soft tissue envelope [3,5,11,12]. These injuries require anatomic reduction, but a balance between fracture reduction and extensive soft tissue dissection must be maintained [5]. Excessive soft tissue stripping for osseous exposure can result in dehiscence, infection, and nonunion [3,5,11,12].

Indirect reduction techniques with percutaneous fixation have been developed in an attempt to decrease the potential complications seen with open reduction internal fixation for tibial pilon fractures. Percutaneous plating and percutaneous cannulated screw fixation are two surgical options for the management of tibial pilon fractures that incorporate the principles of minimal incision surgery in an attempt to protect the soft tissue envelope. These techniques are two of several options for treatment of the tibial pilon fracture, but they are the most appropriate surgical options for the management of these injuries in the high-risk patient.

Percutaneous plating of the distal tibia in tibial pilon fractures maintains arterial vascularity and protects the periosteum and soft tissue from excessive damage secondary to extensive surgical dissection [3,5,12]. In the distal tibia, the plate is most often applied to either the anterior-medial or the anterior-lateral aspect of the tibia. Several commercially produced contoured plates are available for the distal tibia. The authors' preferred method for percutaneous fixation of a tibial pilon fracture in the high-risk patient is through percutaneous plating.

With this technique, a Steinmann pin is first inserted into the posterior tuber of the calcaneus from medial to lateral for skeletal traction, to aid in fracture alignment and reduction. If present, an associated fibular fracture is reduced and fixated first to provide lateral stability and maintain the length of the ankle joint complex. With the assistance of intraoperative image intensification, the main fracture fragments are aligned using percutaneously inserted Kirschner wires, paying careful attention to anatomic reduction of the distal tibial articular surface. Adjunctive use of percutaneously inserted cannulated lag screws may be required, to reduce and stabilize large fracture fragments. Once adequate anatomic alignment is obtained and confirmed through intraoperative image intensification, a plate of appropriate length is selected and inserted through a minimum incision distal to the medial malleolus. A subcutaneous tunnel is created through this incision and the plate is passed through this tunnel to the appropriate position on the distal tibia. Kirschner wires are inserted in the most distal and proximal screw holes to hold the plate in the correct position on the tibia. Percutaneously, one proximal and one distal screw are inserted into the plate and the reduction is then verified by way of intraoperative image intensification. If adequate alignment is noted, screws are placed percutaneously through the remaining screw holes.

The use of percutaneous cannulated screws for fixation of tibial pilon fractures has also been described. In 2004, Syed and Panchbhavi [11] performed a retrospective analysis of seven patients who had a closed distal tibial pilon fracture treated with closed reduction and internal fixation with percutaneous cannulated screws. All seven patients had a displaced tibial plafond fracture without significant comminution or impaction of the distal tibial articular surface. Four of the seven (57%) patients had an associated fibular fracture that was reduced with the use of a dynamic compression plate. The distal tibial fracture was reduced under intraoperative image intensification using manipulation and traction. Fracture reduction was achieved with the use of reduction forceps inserted through minimum-length skin incisions. Guidewires were then inserted into the major fracture fragments and percutaneous cannulated screws used for permanent fracture stabilization were delivered. The investigators reported no soft tissue complications and no nonunions in their small series. They concluded that closed reduction and percutaneous cannulated screw fixation provide sufficient stability in displaced tibial plafond fractures without significant comminution or impaction of the distal tibial articular surface [11].

Summary

Foot and ankle trauma in the high-risk patient presents a surgical dilemma for the foot and ankle surgeon because the possible complications are magnified in this patient population. The use of minimum incisions to reduce fractures and percutaneous delivery of rigid internal fixation provides an alternative to open reduction internal fixation for foot and ankle trauma in the high-risk patient, to reduce the risk for these serious complications. Although the potential exists for less than optimal reduction because of the lack of direct visualization of the osseous injury, percutaneous fixation for foot and ankle trauma provides a safe and satisfactory method of trauma management in the high-risk patient.

References

[1] Padanilam TG, Donley BG. High-risk foot and ankle patients. Foot Ankle Clin 2003;8(1): 149–57.

[2] Seibert FJ, Frankhauser F, Elliot B, et al. External fixation in trauma of the foot and ankle. Clin Podiatr Med Surg 2003;20(1):159–80.

[3] Borg T, Larsson S, Lindsjo U. Percutaneous plating of distal tibial fractures. Preliminary results in 21 patients. Injury 2004;34(6):608–14.

[4] Carr JB. Surgical treatment of intra-articular calcaneal fractures. A review of small incision approaches. J Orthop Trauma 2005;19(2):109–17.

[5] Maffulli N, Toms AD, McMurtie A, et al. Percutaneous plating of distal tibial fractures. Int Orthop 2004;28(3):159–62.

[6] McGarvey WC, Burris MW, Clanton TO, et al. Calcaneal fractures: indirect reduction and internal fixation. Foot Ankle Int 2006;27(7):494–9.

[7] Rammelt S, Amlang M, Barthel S, et al. Minimally-invasive treatment of calcaneal fractures. Injury 2004;35(Suppl):S55–63.

[8] Ray TD, Nimityongskul P, Anderson LD. Percutaneous intramedullary fixation of lateral malleolus fractures: technique and report of early results. J Trauma 1994;36(5):669–75.

[9] Schepers T, Schipper IB, Vogels LM, et al. Percutaneous treatment of displaced intra-articular calcaneal fractures. J Orthop Sci 2007;12(1):22–7.

[10] Stulik J, Stehlik J, Rysavy M, et al. Minimally-invasive treatment of intra-articular fractures of the calcaneum. J Bone Joint Surg Br 2006;88(12):1634–41.

[11] Syed MA, Panchbhavi VK. Fixation of tibial pilon fractures with percutaneous cannulated screws. Injury 2004;35(3):284–9.

[12] Toms AD, McMurtie A, Maffulli N. Percutaneous plating of the distal tibia. J Foot Ankle Surg 2004;43:199–203.

[13] Marcinko DE, Elleby DH. Digital fractures and dislocations. In: Scurran BL, editor. Foot and ankle trauma. 2nd edition. New York: Churchill Livingstone; 1996. p. 353–65.

[14] Spector F, Karlin J, Scurran BL. Lesser metatarsal fractures: incidence, management, and review. J Am Podiatry Assoc 1984;74(6):259–64.

[15] Kirchwehm WW, Figura MA, Binning TA, et al. Fractures of internal metatarsals. In: Scurran BL, editor. Foot and ankle trauma. 2nd edition. New York: Churchill Livingstone; 1996. p. 393–417.

[16] Rammelt S, Heineck J, Zwipp H. Metatarsal fractures. Injury 2004;35(Suppl 2):S77–86.

[17] Sanders R. Fractures of the midfoot and forefoot. In: Mann RA, Coughlin MJ, editors. Surgery of the foot and ankle. St. Louis (MO): Mosby; 1999. p. 1574–605.

[18] Schuberth JM, Patel D. Fractures of the first metatarsal. In: Scurran BL, editor. Foot and ankle trauma. 2nd edition. New York: Churchill Livingstone; 1996. p. 367–92.

[19] Ahmed A, Espley AJ. Fractures of the metatarsals: management of complicated injuries with a simple traction device. Injury 1998;19(5):345–9.

[20] Donahue MP, Manoli A II. Technical tip: transverse percutaneous pinning of metatarsal neck fractures. Foot Ankle Int 2004;25(6):438–9.

[21] Clapper MF, O'Brien TJ, Lyons PM. Fractures of the fifth metatarsal. Analysis of a fracture registry. Clin Orthop Relat Res 1995;315:238–41.

[22] Munro RG. Fractures of the base of the fifth metatarsal. Can Assoc Radiol J 1989;40(5):260–1.

[23] Theodorou DJ, Theodorou SJ, Kakitsubata Y, et al. Fractures of proximal portion of fifth metatarsal bone: anatomic and imaging evidence of a pathogenesis of avulsion of the plantar aponeurosis and the short peroneal muscle tendon. Radiology 2003;226(3):857–65.

[24] Dameron TB Jr. Fractures and anatomical variations of the proximal portion of the fifth metatarsal. J Bone Joint Surg Am 1975;57(6):788–92.

[25] Egol K, Walsh M, Rosenblatt K, et al. Avulsion fractures of the fifth metatarsal base: a prospective outcome study. Foot Ankle Int 2007;28(5):581–3.

[26] Vorlat P, Achtergael W, Haentjens P. Predictors of outcome of non-displaced fractures of the base of the fifth metatarsal. Int Orthop 2007;31(1):5–10.

[27] Husain ZS, DeFronzo DJ. A comparison of bicortical and intramedullary screw fixations of Jones' fractures. J Foot Ankle Surg 2002;41(3):146–53.

[28] Roukis TS, Granger D, Zgonis T. A simple technique for performing percutaneous fixation of fifth metatarsal base fractures. J Am Podiatr Med Assoc 2007;97(3):244–5.

[29] Lawrence SJ, Botte MJ. Foot fellow's review: Jones' fractures and related fractures of the proximal fifth metatarsal. Foot Ankle 1993;14(6):358–65.

[30] Kavanaugh JH, Brower TD, Mann RV. The Jones fracture revisited. J Bone Joint Surg Am 1978;60(6):776–82.

[31] Mologne TS, Lundeen JM, Clapper MF, et al. Early screw fixation versus casting in the treatment of acute Jones fractures. Am J Sports Med 2005;33(7):970–5.

[32] Konkel KF, Menger AG, Retzlaff SA. Non-operative treatment of fifth metatarsal fractures in an orthopaedic suburban private multi-specialty practice. Foot Ankle Int 2005;26(9):704–7.

[33] Porter DA, Duncan M, Meyer SJ. Fifth metatarsal Jones fracture fixation with a 4.5-mm cannulated stainless steel screw in the competitive and recreational athlete: a clinical and radiographic evaluation. Am J Sports Med 2005;33(5):726–33.

[34] Arangio GA. Proximal diaphyseal fractures of the fifth metatarsal (Jones' fracture): two cases treated by cross-pinning with review of 106 cases. Foot Ankle 1983;3(5):293–6.

[35] Grivas TB, Vasiliadis ED, Koufopoulos G, et al. Midfoot fractures. Clin Podiatr Med Surg 2006;23(2):323–41.

[36] Hunter JC, Sangeorzan BJ. A nutcracker fracture: cuboid fracture with an associated avulsion fracture of the tarsal navicular. AJR Am J Roentgenol 1996;166(4):888.

[37] Weber M, Locher S. Reconstruction of the cuboid in compression fractures: short to midterm results in twelve patients. Foot Ankle Int 2002;23(11):1008–13.

[38] Sangeorzan BJ, Swiontkowski MF. Displaced fractures of the cuboid. J Bone Joint Surg Br 1990;72(3):376–8.

[39] Marshall P, Hamilton WG. Cuboid subluxation in ballet dancers. Am J Sports Med 1992;20(2):169–75.

[40] Everson LI, Galloway HR, Shuh JS, et al. Cuboid subluxation. Orthopedics 1991;14(9):1044–8.

[41] Drummond DS, Hastings DE. Total dislocation of the cuboid bone. J Bone Joint Surg Br 1969;51(4):716–8.

[42] Hermel MB, Gershon-Cohen J. The nutcracker fracture of the cuboid by indirect violence. Radiology 1953;60(6):850–4.

[43] Pinney SJ, Sangeorzan BJ. Fractures of the tarsal bones. Orthop Clin North Am 2001;32(1):41–53.

[44] Main BJ, Jowett RL. Injuries of the midtarsal joint. J Bone Joint Surg Br 1975;57(1):89–97.

[45] Phillips RD. Dysfunction of the peroneus longus after fracture of the cuboid. J Foot Surg 1985;24(2):99–102.

[46] Ebraheim NA, Haman ST, Lu J, et al. Radiographic evaluation of the calcaneocuboid joint: a cadaver study. Foot Ankle Int 1999;20(3):178–81.

[47] Solan MC, Moorman CT III, Miyamato RG, et al. Ligamentous restraints of the second tarsometatarsal joint: a biomechanical evaluation. Foot Ankle Int 2001;22(8):637–41.

[48] DeLee JC. Fractures and dislocations of the foot. In: Mann RA, Coughlin MJ, editors. Surgery of the foot and ankle, vol. 2. 6th edition. St. Louis (MO): Mosby-Year Book; 1993. p. 1465–503.

[49] Beaman DN, Roeser WM, Holmes JR, et al. Cuboid stress fractures: a report of two cases. Foot Ankle 1993;14(9):525–8.

[50] Eastaugh-Waring SJ, Saleh M. The management of a complex midfoot fracture with circular external fixation. Injury 1994;25(1):61–3.

[51] Aitken AP, Poulson D. Dislocation of the tarsometatarsal joint. J Bone Joint Surg Am 1963;45:246–60.

[52] Desmond EA, Chou LB. Current concepts review: Lisfranc injuries. Foot Ankle 2006;27(8):653–60.

[53] Buzzard BM, Briggs BS. Surgical management of the acute tarsometatarsal fracture dislocations in the adult. Clin Orthop Relat Res 1998;353:125–33.

[54] Philbin T, Rosenberg G, Sferra JJ. Complications of missed or untreated Lisfranc injuries. Foot Ankle Clin 2003;8(1):61–71.

[55] Myerson MS, Fisher RT, Burgess AR, et al. Fracture dislocations of the tarsometatarsal joints: end results correlated with pathology and treatment. Foot Ankle 1986;6(5):225–42.

[56] Goossens M, De Stoop N. Lisfranc's fracture-dislocations: etiology, radiology and results of treatment. A review of 20 cases. Clin Orthop Relat Res 1983;176:154–62.

[57] Adelaar RS. Treatment of tarsometatarsal injuries. In: Adelaar RS, editor. Complex foot and ankle trauma. Philadelphia: Lippincott-Raven; 1999. p. 161–74.

[58] Zgonis T, Roukis TS, Polyzois VD. Lisfranc fracture-dislocations: current treatment and new surgical approaches. Clin Podiatr Med Surg 2006;23(2):303–22.

[59] Hardcastle PH, Reschauer R, Kutscha-Lissberg E, et al. Injuries to the tarsometatarsal joint: incidence, classification, and treatment. J Bone Joint Surg Br 1987;64(3):349–56.

[60] Quenu E, Kuss G. Etude sur les luxations du metatarse. Rev Chir 1909;39:281–336.

[61] Ross G, Cronin R, Hauzenblas J, et al. Plantar ecchymosis sign: a clinical aid to diagnosis of occult Lisfranc tarsometatarsal injuries. J Orthop Trauma 1996;10(2):119–22.

[62] Curtis MJ, Myerson M, Szura B. Tarsometatarsal joint injuries in the athlete. Am J Sports Med 1993;21(4):497–502.

[63] Gissane W. A dangerous type of fracture of the foot. J Bone Joint Surg Br 1951;33(4):535–8.

[64] Peicha G, Labovitz J, Seibert FJ, et al. The anatomy of the joint as a risk factor for Lisfranc dislocation and fracture-dislocation. An anatomical and radiological case control study. J Bone Joint Surg Br 2002;84(7):981–5.

[65] Lu J, Ebraheim NA, Skie M, et al. Radiographic and computed tomographic evaluation of Lisfranc dislocation: a cadaver study. Foot Ankle Int 1997;18(6):351–5.

[66] Mills WJ. Lisfranc injuries. In: Sangeorzan BJ, editor. The traumatized foot. An American Academy of Orthopedic Surgeons monograph series. Rosemont (IL): American Academy of Orthopedic Surgeons; 2001. p. 31–9.

[67] Kuo RS, Tejwani NC, Digiovanni CW, et al. Outcome after open reduction and internal fixation of Lisfranc joint injuries. J Bone Joint Surg Am 2000;82(11):1609–18.

[68] Jeffreys TE. Lisfranc fracture-dislocation. J Bone Joint Surg Br 1963;45:546–51.

[69] Lee CA, Birkedal JP, Dickerson EA, et al. Stabilization of Lisfranc joint injuries: a biomechanical study. Foot Ankle Int 2004;25(5):365–70.

[70] Alberta FG, Aronow MS, Barrero M, et al. Ligamentous Lisfranc joint injuries: a biomechanical comparison of dorsal plate and trans-articular screw fixation. Foot Ankle Int 2005;26(2):462–73.

[71] Lee EW, Donatto KC. Fractures of the midfoot and forefoot. Curr Opin Orthop 1999;10(3):224–30.

[72] Patterson RH, Peterson D, Cunningham R. Isolated fracture of the medial cuneiform. J Orthop Trauma 1993;7(1):94–5.

[73] Brown DC, McFarland GB. Dislocation of the medial cuneiform bone in a tarsometatarsal fracture-dislocation: a case report. J Bone Joint Surg Am 1975;57(6):858–9.

[74] Compson JP. An irreducible medial cuneiform fracture-dislocation. Injury 1992;23(7):501–2.

[75] Doshi D, Prabhu P, Bhattacharjee A. Dorsal dislocation of the intermediate cuneiform with fracture of the Lisfranc joint: a case report. J Foot Ankle Surg 2008;47(1):60–2.

[76] Sanders JO, McGanity PL. Intermediate cuneiform fracture-dislocation. J Orthop Trauma 1990;4(1):102–4.

[77] Sangeorzan BJ, Benirschke SK, Mosca V, et al. Displaced intra-articular fractures of the tarsal navicular. J Bone Joint Surg Am 1989;71(10):105–10.

[78] Luthje P, Nurmi I. Fracture-dislocation of the tarsal navicular in a soccer player. Scand J Med Sci Sports 2002;12(4):236–40.

[79] Torg JS, Pavlov H, Cooley LH, et al. Stress fractures of the tarsal navicular. J Bone Joint Surg Am 1982;64(3):700–12.

[80] Romash MM. Fractures of the navicular and cuboid. In: Adelaar RS, editor. Complex foot and ankle trauma. Philadelphia: Lippincott-Raven; 1999. p. 145–60.

[81] Eichenholtz SN, Levin DB. Fractures of the tarsal navicular bone. Clin Orthop Relat Res 1964;34:142–57.

[82] Bartz RL, Marymount JV. Tarsal navicular fractures in major league baseball players at bat. Foot Ankle Int 2001;22(11):908–10.

[83] Juliano P, Nguyen H. Fractures of the calcaneus. Orthop Clin North Am 2001;32(1):35–51.

[84] Tornetta P. The Essex-Lopresti reduction for calcaneal fractures revisited. J Orthop Trauma 1998;12(7):469–73.

[85] Tornetta P. Percutaneous fixation of calcaneal fractures. Clin Orthop Relat Res 2000;375: 91–6.

[86] Adelaar RS. Complex fractures of the talus. In: Adelaar RS, editor. Complex foot and ankle trauma. Philadelphia: Lippincott-Raven; 1999. p. 65–94.

[87] Gumann G, DaSilva T, Thomas J. Talar fractures. In: Gumann G, editor. Fractures of the foot and ankle. Philadelphia: Elsevier Saunders; 2004. p. 151–211.

[88] Vallier HA, Nork SE, Benirschke SK, et al. Surgical treatment of talar body fractures. J Bone Joint Surg Am 2003;85(9):1716–24.

[89] Sharma H, Syme B, Roberts J, et al. Technique tip: use of an ACL tibial jig for hallux metatarsal joint fusion, tarsometatarsal and talar fracture fixation. Foot Ankle Int 2008; 29(1):91–3.

[90] Bibbo C, Lin SS, Beam HA, et al. Complications of ankle fractures in diabetic patients. Orthop Clin North Am 2001;32(1):113–33.

[91] Hoffer MM. Percutaneous lateral malleolar trans-tibial pin fixation of unstable ankle fractures. J Trauma 1976;16(5):374–6.

[92] Kim SK, Oh JK. One or two lag screws for fixation of Danis-Weber type B fractures of the ankle. J Trauma 1999;46(6):1039–44.

ELSEVIER
SAUNDERS

Clin Podiatr Med Surg
25 (2008) 721–732

CLINICS IN
PODIATRIC
MEDICINE AND
SURGERY

Percutaneous Reduction and External Fixation for Foot and Ankle Fractures

Luis E. Marin, DPM, FACFAS[a,*], Dennis B. McBroom, DPM[a], Gregorio Caban, DPM[b]

[a]Podiatric Medicine and Surgery–36 Months Residency, Palmetto General Hospital,
Marin Foot and Ankle, 3410 W 84th Street, Suite #100, Hialeah, FL 33018, USA
[b]Section of Podiatric Medicine and Surgery, Palmetto General Hospital,
Marin Foot and Ankle, 3410 W 84th Street, Suite #100, Hialeah, FL 33018, USA

External fixation is an extremely versatile means of providing reduction and rigid fixation for complex foot and ankle fractures, especially those with severe soft tissue injuries such as open, comminuted, or infected fracture-dislocations. The greatest perceived benefit of external fixation is the ability to stabilize complex fractures, which have a high complication rate when treated by traditional means, in a manner that optimizes soft tissue management by limiting the need for extensive dissection [1]. The use of external fixation in acute trauma about the foot and ankle must follow the well-established foot and ankle reconstruction tenets of re-establishing anatomic alignment, stabilizing the fracture until healed, and reducing soft tissue strain [2]. The advantage of external fixation over traditional internal fixation methods is not simply the method of stabilization, but the ability to use a completely closed or percutaneous reduction method on the injured osseous structures, which preserves vascularity to the underlying injured osseous and articular structures [3,4]. Additionally, by maintaining a stable soft tissue envelope, external fixation allows additional reduction methods such as "ligamentotaxis," whereby the intact capsular, periosteal, and ligamentous tissues serve as points of fixation for comminuted, displaced, intra-articular fractures, to be performed as reduction tools and definitive means of stabilization [1–3]. Closed or percutaneous fracture reduction followed by external fixation stabilization is not indicated for every foot and ankle fracture-dislocation but rather, is reserved for the high-risk patient in whom other surgical intervention techniques are likely

---

* Corresponding author. 3410 West 84th Street, Suite #100, Hialeah, FL 33018.
E-mail address: drluismarin@hotmail.com (L.E. Marin).

to develop significant soft tissue and osseous complications and the associated potential for developing a nonfunctional foot or ankle. Conditions under which this approach would be indicated include full-thickness soft tissue injury or formal necrosis; patients at high risk for infection, such as the immunocompromised patient; extensive comminution, especially periarticular fractures; compartment syndrome secondary to crush injury with underlying osseous trauma; talar fracture-dislocations; and distal tibial plafond (ie, pilon) fractures in general, but especially in elderly, diabetic, or osteopenic patients. DiGiovanni [5] lists four settings in which external fixation is especially useful, which include (1) obtaining provisional stabilization and realignment in a grossly unstable injury pattern before definitive management; (2) as a means of observing the soft tissues of a severely traumatized or crushed foot and ankle; (3) as supplemental fixation in certain cases of limited internal fixation; and (4) as an intraoperative fracture reduction aid, especially in a comminuted fracture pattern, through the principles of ligamentotaxis.

The use of closed or percutaneous reduction followed by application of a complex external fixation system is a master-level modality with a steep learning curve. Plain film radiographs of the entire lower leg, ankle, and foot are mandatory to assess osseous alignment and deformities fully. CT scans are reserved for fracture pathology involving articular surfaces or segmental defects. The foot and ankle surgeon must be extremely familiar with the actual equipment he/she is intending to use, in addition to the principles and techniques of external fixation. In general, the authors prefer to use mini or small external fixation for isolated forefoot pathology, and circular, ring-type fixation for midfoot, hindfoot, ankle, and tibia fracture-dislocations with the addition of foot stabilization through use of a footplate when combined forefoot pathology exists. If possible, a preconstructed, circular, ring-type external fixator is used. The diameter and number of rings used, the use of connecting rods and working-length mechanisms, and the configuration of the tensioned wires and half-pins are factors that must be considered to aid in reduction and stabilization of the fracture-dislocation [6]. On occasion, it is not possible to prebuild the external fixation, and in these situations it is necessary to build the external fixator around the fracture pathology. Regardless of approach, the external fixator construct and the method for fracture reduction and stabilization must be planned carefully before entering the operating room.

The authors present their approach to percutaneous fracture reduction followed by external fixation stabilization techniques for foot and ankle fracture-dislocations in the high-risk patient through a series of case illustrations about the forefoot, hindfoot, and ankle.

Comminuted metatarsal fractures

Comminuted metatarsal fractures impose the surgical challenge of obtaining anatomic alignment and maintaining stable fixation until healed.

Surgical goals include restoring metatarsal length, weight-bearing parabola, and metatarsal-phalangeal joint alignment. Axially placed, percutaneous Kirschner wires have historically been used to fixate metatarsal fractures; however, this form of fixation is applicable only when a small segment of osseous comminution is present. Conversely, spanning mini external fixation is the treatment method of choice for open and severely comminuted or segmental metatarsal fractures in which infection, bone loss, and malalignment are common [7]. In the authors' opinion, the use of combined axial Kirschner wires and mini external fixation allows for a stable construct and meets the treatment goals.

The authors present a case example of an elderly man who had multiple medical comorbidities, who sustained closed fractures of the fourth and fifth metatarsals and the cuboid, secondary to a torsional injury of his midfoot. The head of the fourth metatarsal was plantarly displaced and the fourth metatarsal-phalangeal joint was dislocated (Fig. 1A, B).

Under local infiltrative anesthesia and monitored anesthesia coverage, the comminuted metatarsal fractures were addressed first. A Kirschner wire was driven antegrade from distal to proximal, engaging the plantar aspect of the base of the proximal phalanx, and advanced into the fourth metatarsal head. A percutaneous incision over the dorsal aspect of the fourth metatarsal neck fracture was performed and a tissue elevator was inserted to reduce the fracture in the transverse and sagittal planes, followed by advancement of the Kirschner wire to the fourth metatarsal base (see Fig. 1C). This procedure was followed by placement of a mini external fixation device with two 3.5-mm half-pins in the distal and proximal portions of the fourth metatarsal, spanning the fracture to provide additional stability and allow use of ligamentotaxis. A mini external fixator was used to stabilize the comminuted fifth metatarsal and the nondisplaced cuboid fracture, with two 3.5-mm half-pins placed in the distal metaphyseal portion of the fifth metatarsal and two 3.5-mm half-pins placed in the anterior-lateral calcaneus. Half-pins were not placed into the cuboid to avoid displacement of the pre-existing fracture in the cuboid and to allow for ligamentotaxis across the fracture to aid in reduction. The mini external fixations to both fractures were then terminally tightened to complete fracture reduction and stabilization (see Fig. 1D, E).

The postoperative course consisted of strict non–weight bearing, with weekly follow-up visits to perform pin site care. The sutures were removed at 3 weeks and the patient was encouraged to perform active ankle range of motion but to remain strictly non–weight bearing. At the 8-week point, radiographs were obtained and revealed osseous healing sufficient to allow removal of the external fixation and Kirschner wire fixation in the office setting. Touch-down progressing to full weight bearing in a removable walking boot occurred over the next 2 weeks, followed by a period of physical therapy focusing on passive range of motion and strengthening. Following completion of physical therapy, the patient was gradually weaned from the

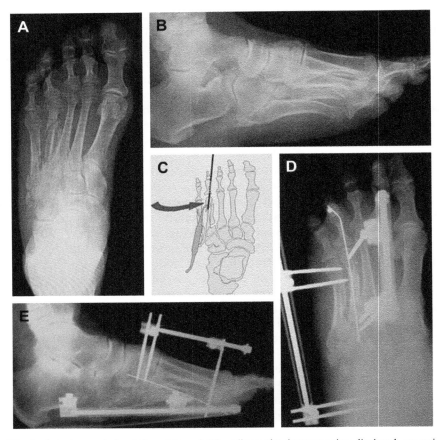

Fig. 1. Anterior-posterior (*A*) and lateral (*B*) radiographs demonstrating displaced, comminuted fourth and fifth metatarsal fractures. (*C*) Use of a tissue elevator to reduce the fourth metatarsal fracture, and insertion of a Kirschner wire for provisional stability. Anterior-posterior (*D*) and lateral (*E*) radiographs following application of mini external fixation devices to the fourth and fifth metatarsal fractures, demonstrating anatomic reduction.

removable walking boot over the next 2weeks, with return to supportive shoe gear.

Multiple metatarsal fractures with associated crush injury

Metatarsal fractures associated with crush injuries of the forefoot are usually associated with severe soft tissue damage and high potential for development of compartment syndrome. As a result of the severe soft tissue and osseous damage, crush injuries require multiple surgical procedures to debride necrotic soft tissues because they declare the true extent of the injury. In the authors' experience, it requires approximately 3 weeks for the soft tissue injury to declare fully the true extent of injury, which is usually much greater than what is obvious on initial examination [8]. The pressure within the pedal compartments should be checked and, when elevated, decompressed through appropriate fasciotomies [9]; any associated fractures should be reduced with the most appropriate and minimally invasive approach available. In this regard, mini external fixation represents a versatile stabilization tool for reduction and stabilization of fractures associated with soft tissue crush injury and compartment syndromes because they span the areas of soft tissue injury and allow frequent wound care without disrupting fracture stabilization, such as would occur with repeated splint applications [7].

The authors' present a case example of a man who had multiple medical comorbidities, who had his foot crushed by a rollover injury from a construction tractor and presented urgently to the emergency department, where he was evaluated. Pedal compartment pressures were evaluated and revealed marked elevation within the interossei, medial, and central plantar foot compartments; in addition, significant pain with motion of the toes demonstrated prolonged toe capillary filling (Fig. 2A). Non–weight-bearing radiographs at the time of presentation revealed first metatarsal-phalangeal joint and sesamoid dislocation, first metatarsal-medial cuneiform dislocation, and fractures of the second, third, and fourth metatarsals distally (see Fig. 2B, C).

Under general anesthesia, the elevated pedal compartments were decompressed using appropriate fasciotomies. Next, the first metatarsal-phalangeal joint and first metatarsal-medial cuneiform joint dislocations were reduced through distal hallux traction and elevation of the first metatarsal base, which were verified under intraoperative image intensification. Two crossed Kirschner wires were placed percutaneously to stabilize the first metatarsal-medial cuneiform joint, followed by application of a mini external fixator using two 3.5-mm half-pins placed into the proximal phalanx and first metatarsal, spanning the first metatarsal-phalangeal joint to maintain reduction and provide stabilization. Using the same technique for percutaneous reduction of metatarsal fractures described previously, Kirschner wires were inserted into the second, third, and fourth metatarsals. The fasciotomy incisions were loosely approximated to limit retraction while allowing reduction of the elevated compartment pressures (see Fig. 2D–H).

This patient's postoperative management mirrored the case example described previously for comminuted metatarsal fractures. Crush injuries often require multiple staged surgical procedures following the index debridement, fasciotomies, and fracture reduction/stabilization. The adjunctive use of hyperbaric oxygen therapy at the authors' institution appears effective at limiting the progression of soft tissue necrosis and begins as soon as possible after the index surgery. Non–weight-bearing passive ankle range of motion is encouraged postoperatively and, once the plantar incisions or wounds fully heal and mature, touch-down weight bearing is permitted with an appropriate gait aid. It is frequently necessary to use

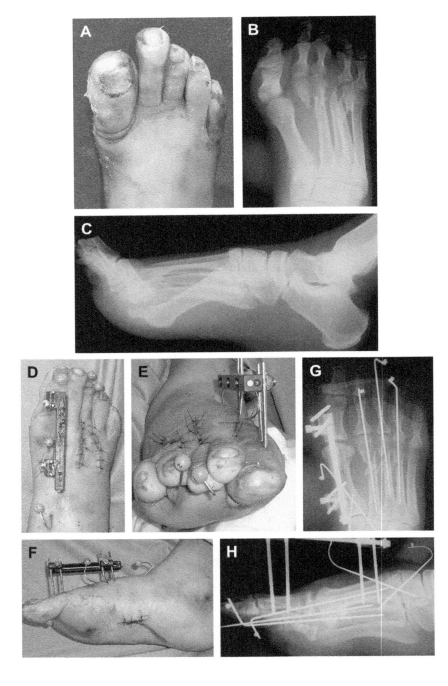

specialized shoe gear and in-shoe orthoses for life to provide a functional result following these devastating soft tissue and osseous crush injuries.

Talar neck fracture-dislocation

Open reduction and internal fixation of talar neck fractures is the current standard of care for operative treatment. These fractures should be regarded as a surgical emergency, and prompt anatomic reduction is mandatory [10]. It seems intuitive that, following anatomic reduction of talar neck fractures, the least invasive stabilization and fracture fixation methods should be considered to limit the potential for further disruption of the arterial supply simply to insert fixation. In the authors' opinion, the use of external fixation to maintain stabilization following anatomic reduction of talar neck fracture-dislocations is beneficial in reducing the incidence of avascular necrosis.

The authors present a case example of an adult man who had multiple medical comorbidities, who sustained a talar neck fracture-dislocation with associated subtalar and talar-navicular joint dislocations following a high-energy injury (Fig. 3). Closed reduction under conscious sedation was performed while the patient was in the emergency department, which successfully reduced the subtalar and talar-navicular joints; however, the talar neck fracture remained displaced.

Under general anesthesia, two parallel transosseous olive wires were carefully placed almost perpendicular to the talar neck fracture. The first transosseous olive wire was placed from the anterior-medial aspect of the talar head across the fracture and exited the posterior-medial tubercle of the talar body. The second transosseous olive wire was placed from the posterior-lateral tubercle of the talar body across the fracture and exited the anterior-lateral aspect of the talar head. These wires were placed while drilling only through bone and then manually tapped through the soft tissues to minimize trauma to the surrounding neurovascular and tendinous structures. Once the placement and orientation of the olive wires were confirmed under intraoperative image intensification, a prebuilt, ring-type external fixation device, consisting of a footplate connected by four threaded rods to an ankle ring, was placed about the foot and ankle. First, the calcaneus was fixated to the footplate by a transosseous wire coursing medial to lateral and tensioned. Next, two converging transosseous wires were placed on the ankle ring proximal to the ankle joint, with care taken to avoid capturing the fibula. At this point, a second converging calcaneal transosseous wire

Fig. 2. (*A*) Anterior-posterior clinical view of the foot following crush injury with associated multiple displaced metatarsal fractures, as demonstrated on anterior-posterior (*B*) and lateral (*C*) radiographs. Anterior-posterior (*D*), en fass (*E*), and lateral (*F*) clinical photographs, and anterior-posterior (*G*) and lateral (*H*) radiographs, following multiple fasciotomies about the forefoot and percutaneous reduction of the metatarsal fractures.

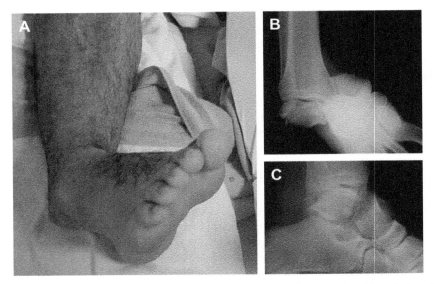

Fig. 3. Anterior-posterior clinical photograph (*A*) and anterior-posterior (*B*) and lateral (*C*) pre-reduction radiographs demonstrating a talar neck fracture-dislocation with associated subtalar and talar-navicular joint dislocations following a high-energy injury.

was connected to the footplate. A midfoot wire was then placed from lateral to medial through the metatarsal bases. A percutaneous incision was made over the dorsal aspect of the talar neck fracture to allow delivery of autologous platelet-rich plasma into the fracture site in an effort to enhance osseous union. The parallel talar transosseous olive wires were loosely fixated anteriorly to a bridge attached to the footplate and posteriorly to the ankle ring. A dual tensioning technique was then performed, whereby both tensiometers were tensioned simultaneously to compress the talar neck fracture gently under direct image intensification. Once fracture reduction was confirmed anatomic, the transosseous olive wires were fixated to the ankle ring and footplate bridge without any further tensioning. The final transosseous wire was placed from converging with the previously placed metatarsal wire on the footplate to complete the construct (Fig. 4).

The postoperative course consisted of early weight sharing with weekly follow-up visits to perform pin site care. At the 8-week point, radiographs were obtained and revealed osseous healing sufficient to allow dynamization of the ring-type external fixation device, to enable vertical pistoning of the threaded rods connecting the footplate and ankle ring. Dynamization was performed for 2 weeks, after which the removal of the external fixation was performed. Touch-down weight bearing progressing to full weight bearing in a removable walking boot occurred over the next 2 weeks, followed by a period of physical therapy focusing on passive range of motion and strengthening. Following completion of physical therapy, the patient was

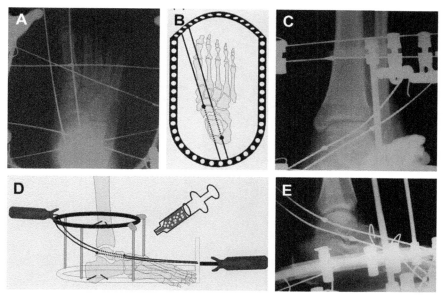

Fig. 4. Anterior-posterior radiograph (*A*) and schematic representation (*B*) of the foot, and anterior-posterior radiograph of the ankle (*C*) following closed reduction and percutaneous stabilization using ring-type external fixation. (*D*) Lateral representation demonstrating application of autologous platelet-rich plasma to the talar neck fracture site. (*E*) Final lateral radiograph demonstrating anatomic reduction and sound stabilization of the talar neck fracture following application of ring-type external fixation.

gradually weaned from the removable walking boot over 2 weeks, with return to supportive shoe gear.

High-risk adult ankle fracture

Adult ankle fractures are usually amenable to open reduction and internal fixation. Acute open ankle fractures and closed ankle fractures with compromised soft tissue envelope, such as a chronic wound or diseased integument, preclude the use of internal fixation, to limit the potential for bacterial colonization that can lead to frank infection. In these situations, the use of external fixation to maintain osseous alignment until healing occurs, rather than using splint or cast immobilization, allows for more rigid stability and makes frequent soft tissue monitoring easier [11].

The authors present a case example of a woman who had multiple medical comorbidities, who sustained a closed bimalleolar ankle fracture-dislocation (Fig. 5A) associated with extensive psoriatic plaques about the lower extremity, except for the medial ankle. The psoriatic plaques had no gross signs of infection, but small fissures were observed that expressed scant serous drainage on compression. After admission for medical

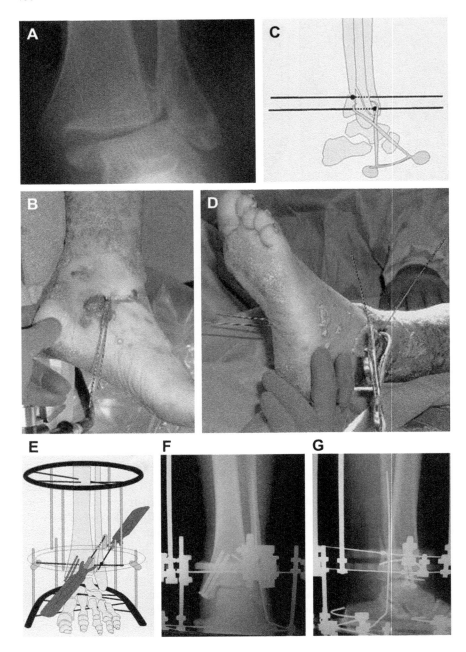

management, a dermatology consult was placed and it was confirmed that the psoriatic plaques, although not grossly infected, were colonized with *Staphylococcus aureus*. To achieve stable fixation of the fibula with the least chance of inducing infection, the surgical technique chosen involved external fixation for the fibular fracture with percutaneous screw fixation of the medial malleolus.

Under general anesthesia, the ankle was reduced by means of closed reduction and periarticular bone reduction forceps were placed anterior to posterior across the fibula to restore proper length and frontal plane alignment. Once this was verified under intraoperative image intensification, the medial malleolus was reduced and fixated using percutaneous placement of 4.0-mm partially threaded cancellous screws (see Fig. 5B–D). Formal stabilization of the fibula was then performed with ring-type external fixation. First, a transosseous olive wire was placed from anterior to posterior at the distal aspect of the fibula, just proximal to the fracture line, at the level of the inferior tibiofibular ligament. A second transosseous olive wire was placed from posterior to anterior just proximal to the posterior spike of the fibular fracture. A ring-type external fixation construct, consisting of a high tibial ring, an ankle ring at the level of the fibular fracture, and a footplate, was assembled using threaded rods. Two converging transosseous calcaneal and proximal tibial wires were placed and tensioned appropriately. The previously placed wires about the fibular fracture were attached to the ankle ring and tensioned with a dual tensioning technique under intraoperative image intensification, followed by removal of the periarticular bone reduction forceps. Once compression was achieved, the transosseous olive wires were attached to the ankle ring without any further tensioning. A transosseous wire was then placed from the distal fibula proximally into the medullary canal for added fibular stabilization. Finally, the midfoot was secured to the footplate with an additional transosseous wire, completing the construction (see Fig. 5E–G).

The postoperative course consisted of early weight sharing with weekly follow-up visits to perform pin site care. At the 10-week point, radiographs were obtained and revealed osseous consolidation sufficient to allow

---

Fig. 5. (*A*) Anterior-posterior radiograph of the ankle demonstrating the displaced bimalleolar fracture. (*B*) Medial intraoperative view demonstrating percutaneous placement of cannulated wires before insertion of cannulated screw fixation following reduction of the medial malleolar fracture. (*C*) Lateral aspect of the ankle demonstrating use of a periarticular bone reduction forceps to reduce and provisionally fixate the fibular fracture, followed by insertion of olive wires. (*D*) Intraoperative photograph demonstrating percutaneous reduction techniques. Note the extensive psoriatic plaques about the lower leg in *B* and *D*. (*E*) Anterior-posterior representation demonstrating application of the ring-type external fixation device and simultaneous tensioning of the olive wires used to stabilize the fibular fracture. Final anterior-posterior (*F*) and lateral (*G*) radiographs demonstrating near anatomic reduction and sound stabilization of the displaced bimalleolar ankle fracture following application of ring-type external fixation.

dynamization of the ring-type external fixation device, to enable vertical pistoning of the threaded rods connecting the footplate and ankle ring. Dynamization was performed for 2 weeks, after which the removal of the external fixation was performed. Touch-down weight bearing progressing to full weight bearing in a removable walking boot occurred over the next 2 weeks, followed by a period of physical therapy focusing on passive range of motion and strengthening. Following completion of physical therapy, the patient was gradually weaned from the removable walking boot over 2 weeks, with return to supportive shoe gear.

Summary

Percutaneous reduction with external fixation of foot and ankle fractures is an effective, minimally invasive means of treating the high-risk patient; however, little has been published about this specific patient population to guide treatment effectively. The authors have presented various cases about the forefoot, hindfoot, and ankle demonstrating the use of these techniques as viable surgical options for those cases in which traditional surgical approaches or techniques pose unnecessary risks for complications that can lead to lower extremity amputation. Percutaneous reduction and external fixation for foot and ankle fractures minimizes the known risks and should be considered an effective approach for the high-risk patient who has foot and ankle fractures.

References

[1] Beals TC. Applications of ring fixators in complex foot and ankle trauma. Orthop Clin North Am 2001;32(1):205–14.
[2] Kaj K. The role of external fixation in acute foot trauma. Foot Ankle Clin 2004;9:583–94.
[3] Paley D, Herzenberg JE. Applications of external fixation to foot and ankle reconstruction. In: Myerson M, editor. Foot and ankle disorders, vol. 2. Philadelphia: WB Saunders; 2000. p. 1135–86.
[4] Seibert FJ, Fankhauser F, Elliot B, et al. External fixation in trauma of the foot and ankle. Clin Podiatr Med Surg 2003;20(1):159–80.
[5] DiGiovanni CW. Fractures of the navicular. Foot Ankle Clin 2004;9:25–63.
[6] Fleming B, Paley D, Kristiansen T, et al. A biomechanical analysis of the Ilizarov external fixator. Clin Orthop Relat Res 1989;241:95–105.
[7] Ziv I, Mosheiff R, Zelgowski A, et al. Crush injuries of the foot with compartment syndrome: immediate one-stage management. Foot Ankle 1989;9(4):185–9.
[8] Myerson MS. Management of crush and soft tissue injuries of the foot. In: Adelaar RS, editor. Complex foot and ankle trauma. Philadelphia: Lippincott-Raven; 1999. p. 175–204.
[9] Andersen CA, Roukis TS. The diabetic foot. Surg Clin North Am 2007;87(5):1149–77.
[10] Juliano PJ, Myerson MS. Fractures of the hindfoot. In: Myerson M, editor. Foot and ankle disorders, vol. 2. Philadelphia: WB Saunders; 2000. p. 1297–340.
[11] Rammelt S, Endres T, Grass R, et al. The role of external fixation in acute ankle trauma. Foot Ankle Clin 2004;9:455–74.

ELSEVIER
SAUNDERS

Clin Podiatr Med Surg
25 (2008) 733–742

CLINICS IN
PODIATRIC
MEDICINE AND
SURGERY

Percutaneous Bone Marrow Aspirate and Bone Graft Harvesting Techniques in the Lower Extremity

Valerie L. Schade, DPM, AACFAS, Thomas S. Roukis, DPM, FACFAS*

Limb Preservation Service, Vascular/Endovascular Surgery Service, Department of Surgery, Madigan Army Medical Center, 9040-A Fitzsimmons Avenue, MCHJ-SV, Tacoma, WA 98431, USA

Autogenous bone transplantation has been the "gold standard" for augmentation of osseous healing [1–4] because it provides all three properties to which allograft bone substitutes strive: osteogenesis, osteoinduction, and osteoconduction. Autogenous bone also eliminates the potential for immunologic incapability and transmission of disease associated with allografts and xenografts [1,2,4–7]. Common donor sites include the sternum, ribs, iliac crest, greater trochanter, fibula, tibia, and calcaneus [2–5]. The iliac crest has traditionally been the most common donor site for cortical and cortical-cancellous autogenous bone graft use in foot and ankle surgery; however, harvesting bone from this area is associated with high morbidity, most notably chronic pain at the donor site. Several studies have reported a 15% incidence of donor site pain lasting longer than 3 months, a 10% incidence of injury to the lateral femoral cutaneous nerve, and a 4% to 10% incidence of superior cluneal and ilioinguinal nerve injury, in addition to superior gluteal artery injury and wound hematoma [1,4,8,9].

Autogenous cancellous bone, in contrast to cortical or cortical-cancellous bone, more rapidly incorporates and revascularizes, leading to more complete repair, and has been shown to be completely revascularized in 2 weeks, compared with 2 months with cortical bone [1,6,10,11]. Autogenous bone

---

The opinions and assertions contained herein are the private views of the authors and are not to be construed as official or reflecting the views of the Department of the Army or the Department of Defense.

* Corresponding author.

E-mail address: thomas.s.roukis@us.army.mil (T.S. Roukis).

0891-8422/08/$ - see front matter. Published by Elsevier Inc.
doi:10.1016/j.cpm.2008.05.001

podiatric.theclinics.com

marrow aspirate and cancellous bone consist of hematopoietic and mesenchymal cell types [12]. Hematopoietic cells differentiate into red and white blood cells, platelets, and macrophages, whereas mesenchymal cells are multipotent and can evolve into several cell types that are involved in tissue repair, depending on the environment to which they are transferred [3]. These cell types include osteoblasts, chondrocytes, fibroblasts, and myogenic cells [12]. Bone marrow is the primary source of mesenchymal cells [3]. Recently, several studies have advocated the use of autologous bone marrow aspirate to augment healing of nonunions, acute fractures, arthrodesis sites, and chronic wounds [1,2,12–14].

For podiatric foot and ankle surgeons, the proximal medial tibial metaphysis and lateral calcaneus offer convenient harvest sites for autogenous bone marrow aspirate and cancellous bone graft, which are now discussed in detail.

Autogenous bone marrow aspirate and cancellous bone graft harvesting from the proximal medial tibia

Autogenous bone marrow aspirate and cancellous bone graft can be harvested from the medial aspect of the proximal tibial metaphysis. This approach allows for obtaining bone material from a zone virtually devoid of neurovascular structures, compared with the approach necessary to access the lateral aspect of the proximal tibial metaphysis [4,15]. Herford and Audia [14] performed a cadaveric study involving 40 lower extremities from 20 cadaveric specimens (10 male, 10 female) with a mean age of 82.1 years (range, 41–97 years) to determine the proximity of neurovascular structures for a medial and lateral approach to the proximal tibia metaphysis and to quantify the amount of cancellous bone obtained for each approach. No significant difference existed in the amount of bone obtained from either approach (medial, 25 mL; lateral, 24.9 mL). This result was similar to that reported by Catone and colleagues [15], who were able to collect a mean of 25 mL of cancellous bone from the proximal tibia. No correlation was found between age and the amount of bone harvested and gender did not produce a significant difference between the amounts of bone obtained [15]. It was found that the lateral approach consistently had branches of the recurrent tibial vessels and nerves passing directly into the area of bone graft harvesting and also violated the anterior compartment of the lower leg. In contrast, the medial approach was a greater distance from nerves and vessels and did not enter any of the lower leg muscular compartments [15]. In contrast to harvesting cancellous bone, no more than 2 mL of bone marrow aspirate should be aspirated from a single site, to maximize the number of alkaline phosphatase-positive, colony-forming units, which are indicative of cells that will differentiate into a mature osteoblastic phenotype. Aspiration of more than 2 mL from a single site results in dilution from peripheral blood, which decreases the bone growth stimulation provided by the cellular tissue within the bone marrow aspirate [11].

The location for portal entry for autogenous bone marrow aspirate and incision placement to obtain cancellous bone graft from the proximal medial tibia has been described in detail by one of the authors (TSR) [11]. This technique consists of the surgeon making a closed fist and placing his/her knuckles at the medial edge of the patellar tendon with the superior surface of the index finger at the level of the proximal aspect of the tibial articular surface. A circle is drawn around the closed fist, the center of which represents a safe zone in which to harvest bone marrow aspirate and cancellous bone graft [11].

For harvesting bone marrow aspirate, an aspirate system (Wright Medical Technology, Inc., Arlington, Tennessee) containing a sharp trocar within a large-bore hollow needle is inserted through the skin at a 90° angle to the medial wall of the proximal tibia and is advanced approximately 0.5 to 1 cm. The combined needle and trocar system is inserted into the bone with a twisting motion and a fair amount of pressure, using the surgeon's dominant hand; or, a Steinmann pin can be used first to gain entry to the cortex, followed by the aspirate system (Fig. 1A). Firmly striking a mallet against the hand piece should be avoided in the proximal tibia to prevent iatrogenic injury or damage to the aspirate system. Once the needle is firmly seated, the trocar is withdrawn and replaced with a 30-mL syringe attached to the aspiration portal (Fig. 1B). The needle is held stationary as the plunger on the syringe is slowly distracted to aspirate between 0.5 and 2 mL of bone marrow aspirate (Fig. 1C). If more volume is needed, the syringe can be advanced deeper from this point and an additional 0.5 and 2 mL of bone marrow aspirate can be obtained. If additional bone marrow aspirate beyond that collected is necessary, the syringe should be removed from the aspiration portal, the trocar reinserted, and the needle withdrawn just enough to redirect it 25° from the original aspiration site in "fan" technique fashion. When the needle is repositioned, the trocar is removed, and the syringe is reattached to aspirate the additional bone marrow, with this process being repeated until a sufficient quantity of bone marrow aspirate has been obtained (Fig. 1D) [11]. One or two staples are used to reapproximate the skin.

For harvesting autogenous cancellous bone graft from the proximal medial tibia, a 1- to 1.5 cm incision is placed through the skin only within the safe zone described earlier [11]. A hemostat is used in line with the incision to dissect bluntly to the underlying bone, followed by insertion of an 8-mm round-core biopsy trephine inserted at a 90° angle to the medial wall of the proximal tibia and advanced 1 to 2 cm deep. With gentle, gradually increasing circular motions, the trephine is retrieved and the graft obtained. Additional cancellous bone graft may be obtained by passing the trephine through the same hole at various angles, as opposed to creating new holes within the medial wall of the proximal tibia, to avoid the possible complications associated with weakening the medial wall of the proximal tibia [16]. Multiple plugs of cancellous bone up to 5 cm in length can be obtained in this manner [11,17]. The bone graft site is typically fully healed within a few weeks without the need for supplemental bone graft substitute

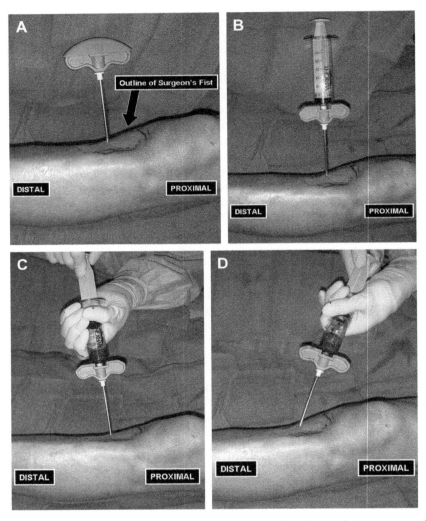

Fig. 1. (*A*) Intraoperative photograph demonstrating the needle and trocar bone marrow aspirate system inserted within the proximal medial tibial metaphysis. Note that the entry site lies within the center of a circle drawn around the surgeon's closed fist, which was placed with his/her knuckles along the lateral aspect of the patellar tendon and the superior aspect of the index finger in line with the proximal aspect of the tibial articular surface. The center of this circle represents a safe zone. The trocar has been removed and the syringe attached to the aspiration portal (*B*) followed by slow and steady aspiration (*C*). Additional autogenous bone marrow aspirate is obtained by reversing the process and redirecting the aspiration system using the technique described above (*D*).

implantation within the osseous void created, although this implantation can be performed if necessary with synthetic bone substitutes that provide structural support (Pro-Dense, Wright Medical Technology, Inc., Arlington, Tennessee). The skin edges of the incision are reapproximated with a single vertical mattress suture of 2-0 nylon and metallic skin staples.

Care must be taken to perform autogenous bone graft harvest from the proximal tibia carefully because the incidence of fracture with proximal tibial harvesting ranges from 0% to 12% and occurs most commonly with harvest of structural cortical-cancellous grafts at the metaphyseal-diaphyseal junction [6,17,18]. Geideman and colleagues [1] performed a retrospective review on 155 patients (90 male, 65 female) with a mean age of 41 years (range, 17–76 years). Although no direct measurements of bone graft obtained were consistently recorded, some operative reports showed that up to 30 cm^2 were obtained. An incidence of one (0.6%) postoperative infection, three (2%) incisional dysesthesias (which resolved before 3 months), and no cases of discomfort by 3 weeks postoperative was reported. Most of these grafts were obtained from a lateral approach, which was the only operative technique described. Whitehouse and colleagues [2] reported the results of harvested bone from the proximal lateral tibia in 131 patients (78 female, 53 male) with a mean age of 53 years (range, 20–82 years) and a mean follow-up of 28 months (range, 3–69 months). Eight (5.4%) patients had immediate transient postoperative anesthesia, 5 (4%) had occasional pain at the donor site, and 1 (0.7%) developed a superficial wound infection [2]. O'Keeffe and colleagues [9] harvested bone graft from the proximal tibia in 230 patients with a mean follow-up of 20.4 months (range, 4–65 months). Results indicated one (0.4%) undisplaced fracture of the tibial eminence, one (0.4%) hematoma, and one (0.4%) superficial wound infection. Lezcano and colleagues [17] performed a retrospective review of 33 patients who had autogenous cancellous bone graft harvested from the proximal medial tibia using a trephine as described here. The investigators reported no major complications at the donor site and two cases of local infection and unaesthetic scar attributable to the lack of soft tissue coverage over the medial tibial metaphysis. They concluded that the medial approach to harvest autogenous cancellous bone grafts from the proximal tibia with a trephine was simple, safe, and predictable [17]. All of these studies reported results from grafts obtained with an open approach, as opposed to a percutaneous approach as described here.

Technique for autogenous bone marrow aspirate and cancellous bone graft harvesting from the lateral calcaneus

Autogenous bone marrow aspirate and cancellous bone graft is most often harvested from the lateral aspect of the calcaneus because of the ease of accessibility and dependable healing [6]. The open structure of the interior calcaneus provides a large endosteal surface with ample amounts of bone marrow, which facilitates diffusion, early vessel ingrowth, and rean-astomosis, and provides an abundance of pleuripotential cells, giving bone marrow aspirate and cancellous graft obtained from the calcaneus excellent osteogenic potential [1,6].

A simple and accurate technique the senior author (TSR) uses for iden-tifying the center of the posterior third of the calcaneus is for the surgeon to place his/her thumb on the origin of the plantar fascia and the index fin-ger of the same hand on the insertion of the Achilles tendon, which creates a semicircle of the surgeon's hand [11,18]. This semicircle is completed with an imaginary line over the lateral aspect of the calcaneus (Fig. 2A) [11,18]. A point marked midway on this line denotes the location for insertion of an 8-mm trephine (Fig. 2B) [11,18]. This location is posterior and inferior to the sural nerve, which courses anterior-lateral to the lesser saphenous vein along the lateral border of the Achilles tendon at the level of the ankle, after which it curves distally approximately 1 to 1.5 cm inferior to the tip of the fibula, and is situated directly within the dense rim of trabecular bone at the posterior third of the calcaneus [5,7,11,18,19].

For harvesting autogenous bone marrow aspirate from the lateral calca-neus, the aspirate system (Wright Medical Technology, Inc., Arlington, Ten-nessee) and technique is the same as that described for the proximal medial tibial metaphysis (Fig. 3A). Alternatively, a medial approach can be used, but this approach does tend to cause more bleeding postoperatively and to be more painful because of the penetration through the abductor hallucis muscle origin site and thicker periosteum about the medial calcaneal wall (Fig. 3B).

For harvesting cancellous bone graft, the landmark for incision place-ment is located as described earlier. A 1.0- to 1.5-cm linear incision is placed through the skin only within the relaxed skin tension lines. A hemostat is used in line with the incision to dissect bluntly to the lateral wall of the cal-caneus. An 8-mm, round-core, biopsy trephine is then inserted at a 90° angle to the lateral wall of the calcaneus. The trephine is passed through the lat-eral wall and into the posterior aspect of the body of the calcaneus until it abuts the medial cortex. This positioning is verified by palpating the medial wall of the calcaneus with the non-dominant hand [18]. Contrary to a previ-ously published study [8], it is not advisable to penetrate the medial cortex of the calcaneus to avoid damage and scar tissue formation about the medial neurovascular and tendinous structures [5,19]. With gentle, gradually in-creasing circular motions, the trephine is retrieved from the wound. Addi-tional cancellous bone graft may be obtained by passing the trephine through the same hole at various angles for the reasons described earlier (Fig. 4A) [5,18]. Alternatively, a small cortical window can be created with hand instrumentation and the cancellous bone retrieved with a curette (Fig. 4B). The cortical window can either be replaced or used at the target site for structural support (Fig. 4C). Regardless of technique, the bone graft harvest site is typically fully healed within a few weeks without the need for

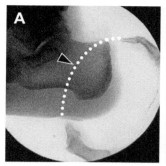
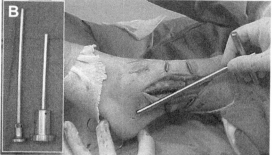

Fig. 2. (*A*) Intraoperative image intensification view of the technique used to identify the proper insertion site to gain access to the lateral aspect of the calcaneus. Note that the thumb of the surgeon's hand is placed on the origin of the plantar fascia and the index finger is placed on the insertion of the Achilles tendon, which creates a semicircle. Continuation of the semicircle (*dotted line*) identifies the ideal location to gain access to the calcaneus (*arrowhead*). (*B*) Intraoperative photograph demonstrating the incision and 8-mm round-core biopsy trephine instrumentation used to harvest autogenous cancellous bone graft from the lateral aspect of the calcaneus.

supplemental bone graft substitute, although allograft bone or synthetic material (Pro-Dense, Wright Medical Technology, Inc., Arlington, Tennessee) can be used to fill the void, further aide in osseous healing, and provide structural support (Fig. 4D). The skin edges of the incision are reapproximated with a single vertical mattress suture of 2-0 nylon and metallic skin staples.

Biddinger and colleagues [8] found that up to three cylinders of bone graft can be obtained with an 8-mm trephine through this technique, using separate portals of entry through the skin and calcaneus for each pass of the trephine. DiDomenico and Haro [7] found that using a percutaneous

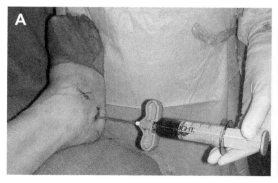
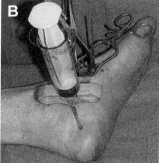

Fig. 3. Intraoperative photograph demonstrating harvest of autogenous bone marrow aspirate from the lateral (*A*) and medial (*B*) aspects of the calcaneus.

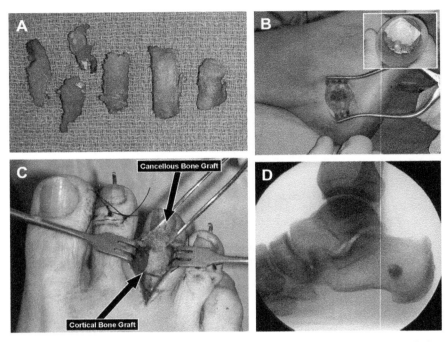

Fig. 4. (*A*) Intraoperative photograph demonstrating the volume of cancellous bone graft that can be obtained with the use of an 8-mm round-core biopsy trephine. (*B*) Intraoperative photograph demonstrating open harvest of cortical-cancellous bone graft from the lateral aspect of the calcaneus, which was used (*C*) to fill a large osseous defect within the third toe following resection of osteomyelitis treated in staged fashion. Note that the cortical aspect of the graft is used to provide structural support and the cancellous bone to provide rapid incorporation. (*D*) Intraoperative image intensification lateral view of the calcaneus following injection of synthetic bone graft substitute (Pro-Dense, Wright Medical Technology, Inc., Arlington, Tennessee) to "back-fill" the bone graft site. Note the location of the harvest site.

technique to harvest bone from the calcaneus with a curette through a drill hole produced 3 to 5 cm^2 of cancellous bone.

Mahan [5,19] performed 25 calcaneal grafts, 7 of which were performed using trephine techniques similar to those described earlier, whereas the others used a segmental approach or a combination of the two methods. The mean time to radiographic consolidation was 8.9 weeks (range, 8–12 weeks) with a mean of 8.9 weeks non–weight bearing (range, 6–12 weeks). One transient peroneal tendonitis lasting a few weeks and one transient neuritis of the posterior calcaneal branch of the sural nerve were noted. All donor sites healed with no infections. Unfortunately, these findings were not reported in such a way that one could differentiate among the three techniques used to harvest calcaneal bone graft [5]. Biddinger and colleagues [8] reported results for the percutaneous trephine harvesting technique on 17 patients (12 female, 5 male) with a mean age of 46.5 years (range, 17–70 years) for a mean follow-up period of 7 months (range, 4–16 months). Three patients (18%) had mild intermittent incisional discomfort, 1 (6%) had local numbness along the distribution of the lateral calcaneal nerve, and 1 (6%) needed minor padding when wearing strapped shoes only. No incidence of hypertrophic scarring, heterotopic ossification, vascular injury, fracture, or collapse was reported [8].

Summary

The proximal medial tibial metaphysis and the lateral calcaneus are excellent sources of autogenous bone marrow aspirate and cancellous bone graft and the many pleuripotential cells contained. Bone marrow aspirate can be directly applied to the desired defect, centrifuged to condense the osteoprogenitor and mesenchymal stem cells, or mixed with autogenous bone graft or allograft bone material. The techniques described here are short procedures that are simple to perform, easily reproduced, and associated with low morbidity and financial cost, making them an ideal adjuvant to enhance soft tissue and osseous healing in high-risk patients.

References

[1] Geideman W, Early JS, Brodsky J. Clinical results of harvesting autogenous cancellous graft from the ipsilateral proximal tibia for use in foot and ankle surgery. Foot Ankle Int 2004; 25(7):451–5.

[2] Whitehouse MR, Lankester BJ, Winson IG, et al. Bone graft harvest from the proximal tibia in foot and ankle arthrodesis surgery. Foot Ankle Int 2006;27(11):913–6.

[3] Smiler D, Soltan M. Bone marrow aspiration: technique, grafts, and reports. Implant Dent 2006;15(3):229–35.

[4] Alt V, Nawab A, Seligson D. Bone grafting from the proximal tibia. J Trauma 1999;47(3): 555–7.

[5] Mahan KT. Calcaneal donor bone grafts. J Am Podiatr Med Assoc 1994;84(1):1–9.

[6] Mendicino RA, Leonhart E, Shromoff P. Techniques for harvesting autogenous bone grafts in the lower extremity. J Foot Ankle Surg 1996;35(5):428–35.

[7] DiDomenico LA, Haro AA III. Percutaneous harvest of calcaneal bone graft. J Foot Ankle Surg 2006;45(2):131–3.

[8] Biddinger KR, Komenda GA, Schon LC, et al. A new modified technique for harvest of calcaneal bone grafts in surgery on the foot and ankle. Foot Ankle Int 1998;19(5):322–6.

[9] O'Keeffe RM, Riemer BL, Butterfield SL. Harvesting of autogenous cancellous bone graft from the proximal tibial metaphysis. J Orthop Trauma 1991;5(4):469–74.

[10] van Damme PA, Merkx MA. A modification of the tibial bone-graft-harvesting technique. Int J Oral Maxillofac Surg 1996;25(5):346–8.

[11] Schweinberger MH, Roukis TS. Percutaneous autologous bone marrow harvest from the calcaneus and proximal tibia: surgical technique. J Foot Ankle Surg 2007;46(5):411–4.

[12] Roukis T, Zgonis T, Tiernan B. Autologous platelet-rich plasma for wound and osseous healing: a review of the literature and commercially available products. Adv Ther 2006; 23(2):218–37.

[13] Hernigou P, Mathieu G, Poignard A, et al. Percutaneous autologous bone-marrow grafting for non-unions: surgical technique. J Bone Joint Surg Am 2006;88(Suppl. 1, Pt 2):S322–7.

[14] Herford AS, Audia F. Medial approach for tibial bone graft: anatomic study and clinical technique. J Oral Maxillofac Surg 2003;61(3):358–61.

[15] Catone GA, Reimer BL, McNeir D, et al. Tibial autogenous cancellous bone as an alternative donor site in maxillofacial surgery: a preliminary report. J Oral Maxillofac Surg 1992; 50(12):1258–63.

[16] Blakemore NE. Fractures at cancellous bone graft donor sites. Injury 1983;14(Suppl. 1): S519–22.

[17] Lezcano FJ, Cagigal BP, Cantera JM, et al. Technical note: medial approach for proximal tibia bone graft using a manual trephine. Oral Surg Oral Med Oral Pathol Oral Radiol Endod 2007;104(1):11–7.

[18] Roukis TS. A simple technique for harvesting autogenous bone grafts from the calcaneus. Foot Ankle Int 2006;27(11):998–9.

[19] Mahan KT. Reply to: a new modified technique for harvest of calcaneal bone graft in surgery on the foot and ankle. Foot Ankle Int 1999;20(1):68.

ELSEVIER
SAUNDERS

Clin Podiatr Med Surg
25 (2008) 743

CLINICS IN
PODIATRIC
MEDICINE AND
SURGERY

Current Concepts and Techniques
in Foot and Ankle Surgery

ELSEVIER
SAUNDERS

Clin Podiatr Med Surg
25 (2008) 745–753

CLINICS IN
PODIATRIC
MEDICINE AND
SURGERY

Use of Circular External Fixation for Combined Subtalar Joint Fusion and Ankle Distraction

Thomas Zgonis, DPM, FACFAS[a],*,
John J. Stapleton, DPM, AACFAS[b],
Thomas S. Roukis, DPM, FACFAS[c]

[a]Podiatry Division, Department of Orthopaedics, The University of Texas Health Science
Center at San Antonio, 7703 Floyd Curl Drive/MCS 7776, San Antonio, TX 78229, USA
[b]Foot and Ankle Surgery, VSAS Orthopaedics, Lehigh Valley Hospital, Cedar Crest Campus,
Allentown, PA, USA
[c]Limb Preservation Service, Vascular/Endovascular Surgery Service, Department of Surgery,
Madigan Army Medical Center, 9040-A Fitzsimmons Avenue, MCHJ-SV, Tacoma, WA
98431, USA

Surgical management of combined symptomatic ankle and subtalar joint arthrosis in a young, active individual is a challenge. Tibiotalocalcaneal arthrodesis is the standard treatment of end-stage posttraumatic arthrosis affecting the ankle and subtalar joint after failure of conservative management [1]. Unlike the hip and knee, the ankle and subtalar joint are rarely affected by primary degenerative joint disease [2]. Rather, trauma is the most common cause for arthrosis of the ankle and subtalar joint [2,3]. As a result, the younger, more active patient is typically affected with severe arthrosis of the ankle and subtalar joint. To date, the treatment options for end-stage posttraumatic arthrosis of the ankle and subtalar joint are double arthrodesis or subtalar joint arthrodesis combined with an endoprosthesis of the ankle joint. However, the literature supports a tibiotalocalcaneal arthrodesis in the younger, more active patient despite the potential complications associated with the procedure [4]. Endoprostheses of the ankle have not performed well in younger, active patients who have severe arthrosis, and many surgeons advise that their use be limited to patients who have light physical demands [5,6]. Joint distraction (ie, arthrodiastasis) offers another treatment option for stiff, painful joints secondary to posttraumatic arthrosis [7–15].

---

* Corresponding author.
E-mail address: zgonis@uthscsa.edu (T. Zgonis).

0891-8422/08/$ - see front matter © 2008 Elsevier Inc. All rights reserved.
doi:10.1016/j.cpm.2008.05.012   *podiatric.theclinics.com*

Tibiotalocalcaneal arthrodesis has been fraught with high rates of complications, with nonunion in up to 60% and infection rates in up to 25% [4,16–19]. Different techniques for a tibiotalocalcaneal arthrodesis have been described using crossed screws, blade plate, external fixation, and intramedullary nail. Currently, with the advent of new intramedullary nails that offer internal compression, the rates of fusion have improved [4,20]. Despite the improvement in fusion rates, the rates of surgical complications remain high with intramedullary implants [1,4,20]. Despite advances in internal and external fixation, a tibiotalocalcaneal arthrodesis is considered a salvage procedure and is used cautiously in primary reconstructive cases. A successful tibiotalocalcaneal arthrodesis can alleviate pain and correct deformity at the expense of joint motion [1,4]. Loss of ankle joint motion will cause persistent alterations in gait that may lead to severe restriction of activity, especially in young, active people [21]. It may also lead to increased stress and deterioration of adjoining joints by ipsilateral or contralateral overloading or compensation [21,22]. Loss of motion is definitive with a successful tibiotalocalcaneal arthrodesis but can also be present preoperatively, secondary to the formation of fibrosis within a posttraumatic joint.

Joint distraction of the ankle can be performed as an alternative to ankle arthrodesis to relieve pain and improve joint function [7–15,23]. Joint distraction, using a circular external fixation frame that bridges the ankle joint, is a new approach in the treatment of severe ankle joint arthrosis. A tensioned wire circular external fixation device allows the surgeon the ability to distract the surrounding soft tissues of a stiff joint, reduce the mechanical stress across a joint, and initiate intermittent intra-articular fluid pressure shift across a joint through axial loading and unloading. Research on osteoarthritic cartilage in vitro by Lafeber and colleagues [24] in 1992 concluded that intermittent hydrostatic pressure applied in the absence of mechanical stress could result in reparative activity by chondrocytes through the production of proteoglycans. Joint distraction by way of external fixation for the treatment of severe osteoarthritis in young patients was first described in 1994 for the hip [25]. In 1995, van Valburg and colleagues [8] published the results of a retrospective study in a preliminary report that included 11 patients, with a mean age of 35 ± 13 years, in which joint distraction was used as an alternative to ankle arthrodesis to treat posttraumatic arthrosis of the ankle. At a mean of 20 months (range, 9–60 months) postoperative, they concluded that short-term joint distraction can be used to delay arthrodesis because none of the patients had proceeded to an ankle arthrodesis. Range of motion improved in 55% of these patients. All 11 patients had less pain and 5 patients had no pain [8]. In 1999, van Valburg and colleagues [15] published the data from the first prospective study on ankle joint distraction with a 2-year follow-up [15]. The investigators confirmed the findings in their previous retrospective study supporting the notion that joint distraction can delay the need for ankle arthrodesis in the presence of severe ankle arthrosis [15]. They found that more than two thirds of the patients improved significantly, as shown by physical examination, functional ability questionnaires, and pain scale [15]. It was also noted that the results were progressive in the second year postoperatively [15]. In 2002, Marijnissen and colleagues [10] published the results of an open prospective study of 57 patients with a mean age of 44 years who were treated with joint distraction as an alternative to ankle arthrodesis [10]. They also published the results of 17 patients who were placed in a randomized controlled study comparing joint distraction with joint debridement [10]. Among the 57 patients enrolled, clinical benefit was apparent in three quarters [10]. The clinical benefit of joint distraction increased over time postoperatively [10]. In the randomized controlled study, joint distraction showed significantly better clinical results than joint debridement alone [10]. Ankle joint distraction is a joint-preserving procedure that can alleviate the pain and joint stiffness associated with severe ankle arthrosis [7–11,13–15].

This article demonstrates the use of a novel approach that combines a subtalar joint fusion with an ankle arthrodiastasis through the use of a tensioned wire circular external fixation frame to prevent or delay the need of a tibiotalocalcaneal fusion.

Indications/contraindications

Young and active patients who experience refractory pain and stiffness to the rearfoot and ankle secondary to combined severe subtalar and ankle arthrosis are suitable candidates for a subtalar joint fusion combined with an ankle arthrodiastasis as an alternative to tibiotalocalcaneal arthrodesis. The authors believe that older patients and sedentary patients are more appropriate for a tibiotalocalcaneal arthrodesis.

Contraindications for surgery include, but are not limited to, the following: arterial insufficiency, neuropathy, Charcot neuro-osteoarthropathy, infection, and psychosocial issues precluding the ability to maintain an external fixation device on the lower limb. Relative contraindications include, but are not limited to, the following: uncontrolled diabetes, ongoing tobacco use, venous insufficiency with chronic venous dermatitis, chronic edema, obesity, osseous ankle deformity, severe ankylosis of the ankle joint, and previous compartment syndrome with residual muscular-tendinous imbalance. Patients who are suitable candidates for joint distraction combined with subtalar joint fusion by way of a circular external fixation frame must display compliance, along with the cognitive ability to understand adequately the procedure, the postoperative course, and the expected outcome with potential risks.

Preoperative planning

A thorough history and physical, with emphasis placed on activity level, is imperative in deciding which patients would benefit from joint distraction versus arthrodesis. The initial traumatic event, associated injuries, and previous course of treatment, if applicable, should be documented. The presence of previous infections, open fractures, and compartment syndrome should be noted. Physical examination should include close evaluation of joint range of motion, the identified symptomatic joints, the associated deformity, and the soft tissue envelope. A gait examination will reveal the patient's ability to compensate for the pain, deformity, or loss of joint motion about the rearfoot or ankle.

Weight-bearing radiographs consisting of foot, ankle, and calcaneal axial views are paramount (Fig. 1). A mechanical axis series should be obtained if lower extremity deformity or a limb length discrepancy is suspected. The physician should evaluate each joint for deformity and arthrosis. CT or MRI can be used to evaluate better the extent of joint arthrosis. MRI or a three-phase bone scan using technetium should be obtained if avascular necrosis or underlying osteomyelitis is suspected.

Noninvasive vascular studies are performed preoperatively if a question exists as to arterial insufficiency based on history or physical examination. A vascular surgery consult should also be obtained preoperatively if studies are equivocal, to prevent further arterial compromise and surgical complication.

The circular external fixation device may be prebuilt outside the operating room before the surgical case, to save valuable anesthesia and operating room time. It is built in a static fashion without hinges and may be constructed with two tibia rings, a footplate, and a half-ring fastened to the footplate and the distal tibia ring. The circular external fixation device should allow room for postoperative swelling while maintaining biomechanical stability.

Operative technique

The procedure is performed under spinal or general anesthesia with the patient positioned in the supine position. Attention is first directed to the anterior-medial ankle, where a 5- to 6-cm skin incision is made just lateral to the tibialis anterior tendon. At this point, an open ankle arthrotomy is performed. Any osteophytes, loose bodies, or exostoses are removed. Subchondral drilling is then performed on accessible areas of the ankle that are denuded of cartilage to promote fibrocartilage formation. Before incision closure, bone wax may be applied over the exostectomy site to limit the potential of osseous regrowth. The ankle is then put through a range of motion to ensure the absence of osseous impingement. If an osseous block is not present but the foot cannot be dorsiflexed to neutral, a percutaneous Achilles tendon lengthening or gastrocnemius recession is performed at this time. Attention is then directed to the lateral aspect of the foot, in which a curvilinear incision is made, beginning below the posterior aspect of the distal fibula and extending toward the base of the fourth metatarsal.

At this point, dissection is carried down to the subtalar joint while reflecting the extensor digitorum muscle belly distally. A lamina spreader is inserted, exposing the subtalar joint. The cartilage of the subtalar joint is then debrided down to bleeding subchondral bone. Allogenic bone graft is then inserted into the arthrodesis site and temporarily stabilized by a large Steinmann pin. Incisions are then irrigated and closed. At this point, the prebuilt circular external fixation device (Ilizarov, Smith & Nephew, Memphis, Tennessee) is positioned on the foot and lower extremity. Opened towels are stacked under the posterior leg and heel until the surgeon can place two fingerbreadths anterior and three fingerbreadths posterior between the frame and the lower leg. The towels can be removed after the foot and leg are suspended by way of the frontal plane wires in the frame. To avoid rotational offset, the frame should be positioned aligning the anterior crest of the tibia with the anterior tabs of the tibia rings. Laterally, the frame should be positioned parallel with the foot, which is positioned 90° to the lower leg. Positioning should be maintained until the wires are tensioned to the frame. Frontal plane wires followed by oblique plane wires are then inserted into the calcaneus, proximal tibia, and distal tibia. These wires are secured to the frame and tensioned by way of a mechanical tensioner in a standard manner. A fine wire is then placed from lateral to medial across the talus and secured by way of a four-hole post to the footplate. At this point, the threaded rods that connect the footplate to the distal tibia ring are loosened, allowing for 5 to 7 mm of joint distraction. The ankle is distracted and the threaded rods are tightened. Compression across the prepared arthrodesis site, with additional ankle joint distraction, is achieved through manual "Russian" tensioning of the talar wire. A second talar wire may be applied at this point for more stability and secured to the footplate. An additional fine wire is placed across the midfoot to prevent an equinus forefoot contracture and to reduce torsional forces from the foot. Intraoperative image intensification is then used to confirm appropriate ankle joint distraction and compression across the arthrodesis site. (Additional ankle distraction can be performed at postoperative visits.) Dressings are then applied and secured within the circular external fixator.

Postoperative management

Postoperatively, the patient is admitted to the hospital floor for pain, edema control, medical observation, and physical therapy. The patient is placed on a patient-controlled analgesic pump for the first 24 hours. Initially, the operative limb is kept elevated for edema control. The neurovascular status of the limb is checked routinely. The patient is instructed by physical therapy to be strict non–weight bearing on the operative limb. The patient is then discharged home or to a rehabilitation service once pain and edema are well controlled and the patient has met the requirements of physical therapy to be non–weight bearing. The authors keep the patient

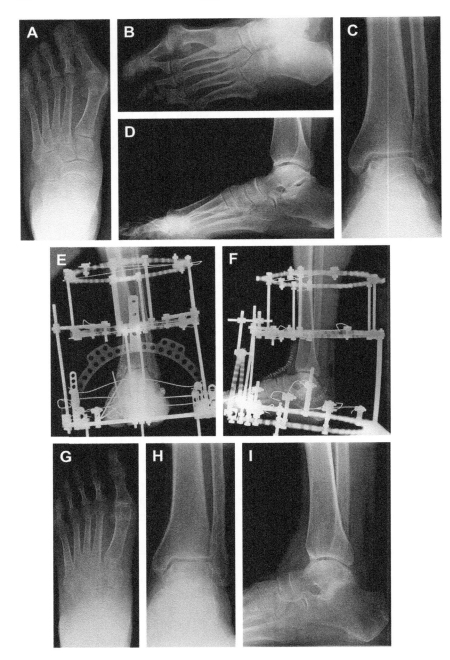

non–weight bearing for the first 10 to 14 days. At 2 weeks postoperatively, the circular external fixation device is modified to add a surgical shoe and the patient is instructed to begin partial weight bearing, progressing to full weight bearing over the next week [26]. The patient is seen every 2 to 3 weeks postoperatively, at which time dressings are performed. Serial radiographs are obtained postoperatively to evaluate the fusion site and to quantify in millimeters the amount of ankle joint distraction. Between weeks 8 and 12, the external fixation frame is removed in the operating room under intravenous sedation and local anesthesia. The patient is then progressed to a walking cast or removable boot for an additional 4 weeks before returning to accommodative shoe gear. Patients return to their normal activities between 4 and 6 months postoperatively.

Discussion

Combining joint compression with joint distraction through the use of a circular external fixation device to achieve a subtalar joint fusion and an ankle arthrodiastasis is a new approach based on sound principles in the treatment of severe arthrosis affecting the ankle and subtalar joint. This treatment option offers hope to the young, active patient who is typically affected with this condition. The authors' rationale is that patient satisfaction, functional outcome, and rate of union are higher for an isolated subtalar joint arthrodesis as opposed to an ankle arthrodesis [27–30]. For this reason, the authors perform a subtalar joint fusion with ankle distraction to minimize the complications that are associated with fusing the ankle. Progression of ankle arthrosis despite joint distraction may be seen on postoperative radiographs but should be correlated with the patient's symptoms. Often, patients experience pain relief and improved function despite radiographs that show progression of the degenerative changes. Also, the literature shows that the clinical benefit of ankle arthrodiastasis is usually cumulative over time [10,23]. For this reason, patients should be educated and encouraged to delay ankle arthrodesis early in the postoperative course if symptoms persist after an ankle arthrodiastasis. The authors speculate

Fig. 1. Preoperative anterior-posterior (A) and oblique (B) foot views and anterior-posterior (C) and lateral (D) ankle views. Note the significant degenerative changes across the ankle, subtalar, and first metatarsal-phalangeal joints. Postoperative anterior-posterior (E) and lateral (F) ankle views showing the bent wire technique for the simultaneous subtalar joint arthrodesis and ankle arthrodiastasis procedures. The osteochondral defect at the medial talar dome was drilled for a fibrocartilage growth. A first metatarsophalangeal joint arthrodesis and a percutaneous tendo-Achilles lengthening were also performed at the time of surgery. Final postoperative anterior-posterior foot view (G) and anterior-posterior (H) and lateral (I) ankle views at 1-year follow-up. Note the repair at the medial talar dome, ankle arthrodiastasis outcome, and complete union at the subtalar joint.

that delaying the need for a joint destructive procedure in a young, active patient could be paramount in an era where advancements to ankle implants are near.

Summary

The authors presented a novel surgical approach for the young and active patient affected with a severe ankle and subtalar joint arthrosis. The authors are currently prospectively reviewing their surgical experience with this procedure and believe that it provides an alternative option for the patient, with potentially promising long-term results.

References

[1] Mendicino RW, Catanzariti AR, Saltrick KR, et al. Tibiotalocalcaneal arthrodesis with retrograde intramedullary nailing. J Foot Ankle Surg 2004;43(2):82–6.

[2] Thomas RH, Daniels TR. Ankle arthritis. J Bone Joint Surg Am 2003;85(5):923–36.

[3] Easley ME, Trnka HJ, Schon LC, et al. Isolated subtalar arthrodesis. J Bone Joint Surg Am 2000;82(5):613–24.

[4] Goebel M, Gerdesmeyer L, Muckley T, et al. Retrograde intramedullary nailing in tibiotalocalcaneal arthrodesis: a short-term, prospective study. J Foot Ankle Surg 2006;45(2): 98–106.

[5] Saltzman CL. Perspective on total ankle replacement. Foot Ankle Clin 2000;5(4):761–75.

[6] Gould JS, Alvine FG, Mann RA, et al. Total ankle replacement: a surgical discussion. Part I. Replacement systems, indications, and contraindications. Am J Orthop 2000;29(8):604–9.

[7] Paley D, Lamm BM. Ankle joint distraction. Foot Ankle Clin 2005;10(4):685–98.

[8] van Valburg AA, van Roermund PM, Lammens J, et al. Can Ilizarov joint distraction delay the need for an arthrodesis of the ankle? A preliminary report. J Bone Joint Surg Br 1995; 77(5):720–5.

[9] Marijnissen AC, van Roermund PM, van Melkebeek J, et al. Clinical benefit of joint distraction in the treatment of ankle osteoarthritis. Foot Ankle Clin 2003;8(2):335–46.

[10] Marijnissen AC, Van Roermund PM, Van Melkebeek J, et al. Clinical benefit of joint distraction in the treatment of severe osteoarthritis of the ankle: proof of concept in an open prospective study and in a randomized controlled study. Arthritis Rheum 2002; 46(11):2893–902.

[11] van Roermund PM, van Valburg AA, Duivemann E, et al. Function of stiff joints may be restored by Ilizarov joint distraction. Clin Orthop Relat Res 1998;348:220–7.

[12] van Roermund PM, Marijnissen AC, Lafeber FP. Joint distraction as an alternative for the treatment of osteoarthritis. Foot Ankle Clin 2002;7(3):515–27.

[13] van Roermund PM, Lafeber FP. Joint distraction as treatment for ankle osteoarthritis. Instr Course Lect 1999;48:249–54.

[14] Chiodo CP, McGarvey W. Joint distraction for the treatment of ankle osteoarthritis. Foot Ankle Clin 2004;9(3):541–53.

[15] van Valburg AA, van Roermund PM, Marijnissen AC, et al. Joint distraction in treatment of osteoarthritis: a two-year follow-up of the ankle. Osteoarthritis Cartilage 1999;7(5):474–9.

[16] Breitfuss H, Muhr G, Monnig B. [Fixation or screws in arthrodeses of the upper ankle joint. A retrospective comparison of 76 patients]. Unfallchirurg 1989;92(5):245–53 [in German].

[17] Miehlke W, Gschwend N, Rippstein P, et al. Compression arthrodesis of the rheumatoid ankle and hindfoot. Clin Orthop Relat Res 1997;340:75–86.

[18] Boobbyer GN. The long-term results of ankle arthrodesis. Acta Orthop Scand 1981;52(1): 107–10.

[19] Muller EJ, Wick M, Muhr G. Surgical management of posttraumatic mal-alignments and arthroses in the ankle. Orthopade 1999;28(6):529–37.

[20] Millett PJ, O'Malley MJ, Tolo ET, et al. Tibiotalocalcaneal fusion with a retrograde intramedullary nail: clinical and functional outcomes. Am J Orthop 2002;31(9):531–6.

[21] Thomas R, Daniels TR, Parker K. Gait analysis and functional outcomes following ankle arthrodesis for isolated ankle arthritis. J Bone Joint Surg Am 2006;88(3):526–35.

[22] Buchner M, Sabo D. Ankle fusion attributable to posttraumatic arthrosis: a long-term follow-up of 48 patients. Clin Orthop Relat Res 2003;406:155–64.

[23] Ploegmakers JJ, van Roermund PM, van Melkebeek J, et al. Prolonged clinical benefit from joint distraction in the treatment of ankle osteoarthritis. Osteoarthritis Cartilage 2005;13(7): 582–8.

[24] Lafeber FP, van der Kraan PM, van Roy HL, et al. Local changes in proteoglycan synthesis during culture are different for normal and osteoarthritic cartilage. Am J Pathol 1992;140(6): 1421–9.

[25] Aldegheri R, Trivella G, Saleh M. Articulated distraction of the hip. Conservative surgery for arthritis in young patients. Clin Orthop Relat Res 1994;(301):94–101.

[26] Roukis TS, Zgonis T. Postoperative shoe modifications for weightbearing with the Ilizarov external fixation system. J Foot Ankle Surg 2004;43(6):433–5.

[27] Haskell A, Pfeiff C, Mann R. Subtalar joint arthrodesis using a single lag screw. Foot Ankle Int 2004;25(11):774–7.

[28] Frey C, Halikus NM, Vu-Rose T, et al. A review of ankle arthrodesis: predisposing factors to nonunion. Foot Ankle Int 1994;15(11):581–4.

[29] Helm R. The results of ankle arthrodesis. J Bone Joint Surg Br 1990;72(1):141–3.

[30] Zgonis T, Stapleton JJ, Roukis TS. Use of the Taylor spatial frame for arthrodiastasis of the ankle joint. Techniques in Foot and Ankle Surgery 2007;6(3):201–7.

ELSEVIER
SAUNDERS

Clin Podiatr Med Surg
25 (2008) 755–762

CLINICS IN
PODIATRIC
MEDICINE AND
SURGERY

Salvage of the First Ray with Concomitant Septic and Gouty Arthritis by Use of a Bone Block Joint Distraction Arthrodesis and External Fixation

John J. Stapleton, DPM, AACFAS[a,b],
Roberto H. Rodriguez, DPM, AACFAS[c],
Luke C. Jeffries, DPM, AACFAS[c],
Thomas Zgonis, DPM, FACFAS[c,]*

[a]*Foot and Ankle Surgery, VSAS Orthopaedics, Lehigh Valley Hospital,
Cedar Crest Campus, Allentown, PA, USA*
[b]*Penn State College of Medicine, 500 University Drive, Hershey, PA 17033, USA*
[c]*Podiatry Division, Department of Orthopaedics, The University of Texas Health Science
Center at San Antonio, 7703 Floyd Curl Drive/MCS 7776, San Antonio, TX 78229, USA*

Concomitant septic and gouty arthritis is a difficult surgical entity for the reconstructive foot and ankle surgeon. Although the association of septic and urate-crystal-induced arthritis has been reported in other locations, the reported cases of salvage of the first metatarsal-phalangeal joint septic gouty arthritis has not been previously reported [1–5]. In this article, the authors present a unique case of an acute gout attack with chronic gouty tophi superimposed with osteomyelitis and septic arthritis. When presented with compromised soft-tissues and significant bone loss to the hallux and first metatarsal, few options remain to achieve salvage in lieu of partial foot amputation. This article discusses the rationale along with the surgical techniques that were used to achieve a successful bone block arthrodesis to prevent amputation in this clinical case scenario.

Case report

A 37 year-old Caucasian male presented to the emergency department at the University of Texas Health Science Center at San Antonio with

---

* Corresponding author.
E-mail address: zgonis@uthscsa.edu (T. Zgonis).

0891-8422/08/$ - see front matter © 2008 Elsevier Inc. All rights reserved.
doi:10.1016/j.cpm.2008.05.014   *podiatric.theclinics.com*

a complaint of relentless pain, redness, swelling, and drainage isolated to his left first metatarsal-phalangeal joint that had began 2 weeks before his presentation and had progressively worsened. He denied previous acute gout attacks to the first metatarsal-phalangeal joint. The patient was initially treated for his chief complaint with a course of oral Amoxicillin for 10 days time without resolution or improvement before arriving to the emergency department. Review of systems revealed concomitant fevers, chills, cold sweats, and episodes of emesis. Past medical history was significant for gastro-esophageal reflux disease and chronic regional pain syndrome that affected the left lower extremity after being involved in a motor vehicle accident. Social history was significant for occasional social alcohol use. Occupational and environmental conditions did not show a risk for lead exposure. Past surgical history was significant for previous left knee arthroscopy for suspected septic arthritis 3 years before his initial presentation. He reported that in the past, there was a concern and suspicion for underlying gout or septic arthritis to the left knee joint because he previously experienced severe pain and displayed signs of inflammation on multiple occasions, but diagnostic joint aspirations and eventual arthroscopy of the knee did not confirm the diagnosis for gout or infection.

Clinically, the patient had stable vital signs. The patient's first metatarsal-phalangeal joint was exquisitely tender on palpation and accompanied by signs of inflammation including erythema, calor, dolor, and edema along with two draining sinuses that revealed an exudate upon expression consistent with chronic gouty tophi. Erythema that was present dissipated immediately with elevation of the extremity more characteristic of gout than cellulitis. Aspirated joint fluid obtained in the emergency department subsequently demonstrated negatively bi-fringent needle shaped crystals under polarized light microscopy representing monosodium urate crystals consistent with the diagnosis of gout. Laboratory findings were remarkable for a serum uric acid of 13 mg/dL and a white blood cell count of 11,100 cells/mL with no left shift and a sedimentation rate of 22-mm/hr.

Foot radiographs demonstrated a well-defined soft-tissue density about the first metatarsal-phalangeal joint extending into the first intermetatarsal space, extensive intra-articular destruction of the first metatarsal-phalangeal joint and overhanging punched out erosions located along the extra-articular peripheral margin of the joint suggestive of chronic gout with possible osteomyelitis and septic arthritis. In addition, radiographs revealed expansile cystic lesions within the first metatarsal head raising suspicion for a neoplastic process. The presentation of gouty tophi consistent with chronic gout presenting with clinical signs of an acute attack with possible infection after only two weeks with no previous history of a gout attack to the first metatarsal-phalangeal joint could not be easily explained, raising suspicion of the possibility of an underlying neoplasm or superimposed infection. The patient was initially referred for magnetic resonance imaging (MRI) as the suspicion for a soft tissue mass such as tumoral calcinosis, possible neoplasm, and superimposed infection needed to be ruled out. MRI was consistent with to-phaceous gouty arthropathy along with superimposed infection. Initial cultures of the joint aspirate acquired in the emergency department were negative for an infectious process. The patient was discharged and managed with indocin and doxycycline by the internal medicine team.

Twelve days after the initial emergency department presentation, the patient was readmitted to the hospital for septic gouty arthritis (Fig. 1). The patient was febrile with a white blood cell count of 20,100 cells/mL and a left shift, C-reactive protein of 272.9 mg/L and a serum uric acid of 11.2 mg/dL. The patient was started on intravenous antibiotics and fluids and then, observed daily. After three days of broad spectrum empiric anti-biotics the patient was afebrile and the white blood cell count was trended down to 13, 400 cells/mL. However, clinical examination of the area showed no signs of improvement as intense inflammatory changes with gouty tophi draining from the sinus tracts were still apparent. On the fourth admission day, the patient was transported to the operating suite for open incision and drainage with resection arthroplasty of the first metatarsophalangeal joint. Without a tourniquet, a linear incision was made over the dorsal-medial aspect of the first metatarsal-phalangeal joint with excision of the dorsal sinus tract. There was an exuberant formation of tophaceous appearing material mixed with purulent drainage about the first metatarsal-phalangeal joint. Evaluation of the articular surface revealed complete obliteration of the articular cartilage and erosive changes noted to the first metatarsal head and phalangeal base. In addition, the tophaceous exudate was noted to infiltrate the surrounding extra-articular soft tissues. All apparent tophaceous material, infected and nonviable soft tissue were meticulously excised. The first metatarsal phalangeal joint was then resected via a sagittal saw until bleeding bone was evident (Fig. 2A, B). The exudate, soft tissue, and

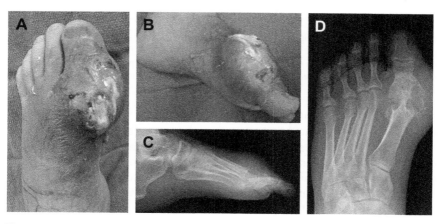

Fig. 1. Anterior-posterior (*A*) and lateral (*B*) clinical photographs, as well as anterior-posterior (*C*) and lateral (*D*) radiographs, demonstrating the significant amount of gouty tophi, cellulitis, erythema, soft-tissue and osseous loss.

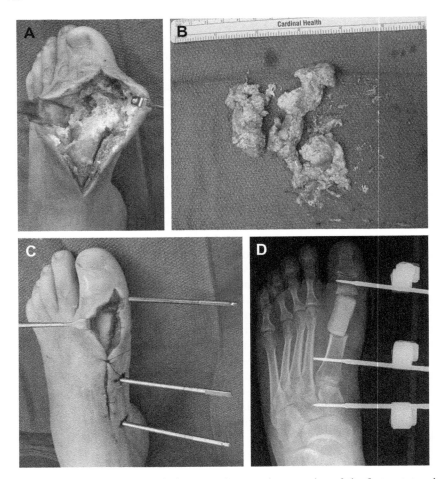

Fig. 2. Intraoperative photograph demonstrating complete resection of the first metatarsal-phalangeal joint (A) and the volume of infected tophi and bone resected (B). Intraoperative photograph (C) and anterior-posterior radiograph (D) following insertion on the polymethyl-methacrylate antibiotic-loaded bone cement spacer and stabilization of the first ray with an external fixation device.

resected bone were sent to both histopathology and microbiology departments for gram stain, acid fast stain, fungal cultures, anaerobic and aerobic culture, and sensitivities. In addition, the exudate was sent for microscopic evaluation under polarized light for confirmation of monosodium urate crystals. After a thorough débridement and joint resection the wound was irrigated with 9 L of normal saline via pulsatile lavage. Hemostasis was then achieved and wet-to-dry dressing was applied to the wound and a posterior splint was applied to the extremity.

Inpatient management continued with empiric parenteral antibiotic therapy pending definitive culture and sensitivities. Intraoperative tissue

and bone cultures were positive for *Staphylococcus aureus* and Propioni-
bacterium species sensitive to oxacillin, vancomycin, erythromycin, clindamycin and doxycycline. Histopathology results demonstrated the presence
of gouty tophi, monosodium urate crystals, poly-morphonuclear leuko-
cytes, and foreign body giant cell reaction. After 5 days of culture-specific
antibiotic therapy, the patient returned to the operating room for revision
surgical débridement, placement of a gentamycin impregnated polymethylmethacrylate cement spacer measuring 3-cm in length, and application
of a uniplane monolateral external fixation device to maintain the length
of the first ray while simultaneously providing immobilization (Fig. 2C,
D). The wound was closed after placement of the antibiotic impregnated
cement spacer.

The patient was subsequently discharged to home on postoperative day
23. Infectious disease care providers ordered 14 days of oral clindamycin
and 4 additional days of parenteral ceftriaxone to complete his antibiotic
regimen. Definitive surgical treatment was deferred until the incision was
healed, edema resolved, and no clinical signs of infection were apparent.
The goal was to leave the antibiotic impregnated cement spacer in for
a minimum of 6 to 8 weeks time if needed.

After an interval of 6 weeks with periodic outpatient monitoring, the
patient was readmitted to the hospital for definitive management. The
patient's surgical procedure began with the harvesting of an autogenous
iliac crest graft from the ipsilateral extremity by the orthopedic service,
removal of the mono lateral connecting bar and extraction of the antibiotic cement spacer. The iliac crest graft was sized with the cement spacer
as a template (Fig. 3A). After placement of the graft, stabilization of the
first ray was achieved using the intramedullary placement of a Steinman
pin across the graft and the application of a 9-hole plate (Fig. 3B, C)
with re-application of the monolateral external fixation device. The
wound edges were re-approximated (Fig. 3D). The patient's postoperative
course was complicated by incision site dehiscence at the 6th week that
necessitated a return to the operative theater for surgical débridement
and soft tissue coverage with a local double advancement rotational
flap. At that time, the external fixation device was removed and the patient was placed into a well-padded short-leg cast and kept nonweight-
bearing. Ten weeks postoperatively from the time the bone graft was
placed the Steinman pins were removed in the office. Nonweight-bearing
was continued for a total of 3 months and then partial weight-bearing in
a surgical shoe was permitted until radiographic healing of the arthrodesis
site was apparent. The patient's radiographs displayed complete osseous
trabeculation across the proximal and distal arthrodesis site at 4 months
postoperatively and was permitted full weight-bearing in a regular shoe at
that point. The patient was refrained from strenuous activities for
2 additional months and discharged at 8 months postoperatively with
no limitations (Fig. 4).

760	STAPLETON et al

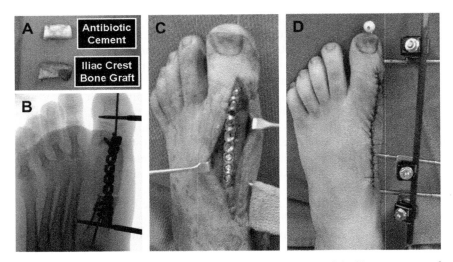

Fig. 3. Intraoperative photograph demonstrating the size and shape of the iliac crest autograft following removal of the polymethylmethacrylate antibiotic-loaded bone cement spacer (A). Anterior-posterior radiograph (B) and clinical photograph (C) following insertion of the iliac crest autograft and application of internal and external fixation. Intraoperative photograph demonstrating primary closure of the incision and use of Steinmann pin and external fixation device stabilization (D).

Discussion

Hyperuricemia is defined as a serum uric acid concentration above 7-mg/dl (420 μmol per L). This concentration is also the limit of solubility for monosodium urate in plasma. At levels of 8-mg per dL (480 μmol per L) or greater, monosodium urate is more likely to precipitate in tissues [6,7]. Although hyperuricemia is a risk factor for the development of gout, the exact relationship between hyperuricemia and acute gout is unclear [2,6–11]. Acute gouty arthritis can occur in the presence of normal serum uric acid concentrations [10,11]. Conversely, many people with hyperuricemia never experience an attack of gouty arthritis [7,8]. Hyperuricemia can have many causes. Serum uric acid levels become elevated in any disorder that results in the proliferation of cells or the excessive turnover of nucleoproteins [2,6–9]. Hyperuricemia can also occur with decreased renal function and in genetic disorders that increase the production or limit the excretion of uric acid. Medications such as diuretics, salicylates, levodopa, and alcohol can limit the excretion of uric acid leading to hyperurecimia [2,6–9].

In this case presentation, primary idiopathic hyperuricemia resulted in the development of tophaceous gout and joint destruction and presented initially with an acute gout attack and a superimposed deep infection. The first step was excluding the possibility of a neoplasm through MRI. The MRI raised the concern for underlying and/or superimposed infection. The

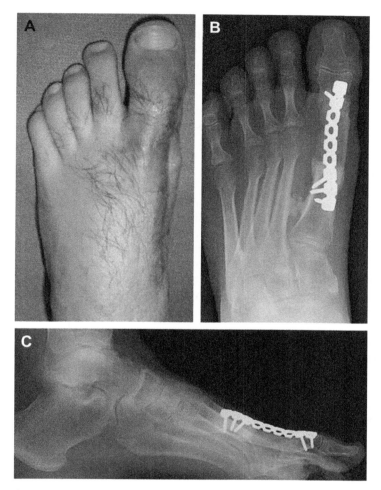

Fig. 4. Final clinical photograph (*A*), as well as anterior-posterior (*B*) and lateral (*C*) radiographs, demonstrating complete soft-tissue and osseous healing with a stable and functional outcome.

patient did not respond well to initial antibiotic treatment. Clinical improvement was not apparent until surgical débridement was initiated. Caution should be used when operating on an acute urate crystal induced arthritis because the potential for vasospasm and gangrene can occur and this should be discussed with the patient. The authors have shown that the surgical management needs to be staged and the timing of surgery is paramount to achieve salvage and prevent complications. In addition, the use of an antibiotic-impregnated cement spacer for the second procedure was advantageous for several reasons: 1) it assisted in stabilizing and maintaining length to the first ray after a large bone resection was performed; 2) it effectively managed the dead space created after the aggressive débridement; 3) it increased the concentration of antibiotics to the affected area; and 4) it re-established a periosteal sleeve for delayed bone grafting. The use of the external fixator was paramount to eliminate motion, decrease the inflammatory response, and to maintain length of the first ray [12,13]. Attention to appropriately obtain joint aspirations, soft-tissue, and osseous cultures for appropriate antibiotic selection cannot be overlooked and the results should be coordinated with an infectious disease specialist to select the most effective antibiotic regimen with the least side effects.

Summary

A stepwise approach to the surgical management of a septic gouty arthritis is essential for salvage. A multidisciplinary team consisting of surgical and medical disciplines was necessary to adequately manage this difficult clinical case scenario. The use of internal and external fixation offered compression and reduced all rotational and torque forces across the arthrodesis site. Finally, the authors believe that medical management of hyperuricemia also needs to be established to prevent future related complications and systemic involvement.

References

[1] Poiraudeau S, Gaudouen C, Dryll A. [Simultaneous septic and gouty arthritis]. Rev Rhum Mal Osteoartic 1988;55(12):1039, [in French].

[2] Ilahi OA, Swarna U, Hamill RJ, et al. Concomitant crystal and septic arthritis. Orthopedics 1996;19(7):613–7.

[3] Salvi A, Rossi M, Balestrieri GP, et al. Septic polyarthritis in chronic tophaceous gout Recenti Prog Med 1991;82(10):527–8.

[4] Schuind FA, Remmelink M, Pasteels JL. Co-existent gout and septic arthritis at the wrist: a case report. Hand Surg 2003;8(1):107–9.

[5] Yu KH, Luo SF, Liou LB, et al. Concomitant septic and gouty arthritis–an analysis of 30 cases. Rheumatol (Oxford) 2003;42(9):1062–6.

[6] Agudelo CA, Wise CM. Gout and hyperuricemia. Curr Opin Rheumatol 1991;3(4):684–91.

[7] Harris MD, Siegel LB, Alloway JA. Gout and hyperuricemia. Am Fam Physician 1999; 59(4):925–34.

[8] Chui CH, Lee JY. Diagnostic dilemmas in unusual presentations of gout. Aust Fam Physician 2007;36(11):931–4.

[9] Villiger PM. [Gout and its differential diagnosis]. Ther Umsch 2004;61(9):563–6 [in German].

[10] Wortmann RL. Gout and hyperuricemia. Curr Opin Rheumatol 2002;14(3):281–6.

[11] Weinberger A. Gout, uric acid metabolism, and crystal-induced inflammation. Curr Opin Rheumatol 1995;7(4):359–63.

[12] Zgonis T, Jolly GP, Blume P. External fixation use in arthrodesis of the foot and ankle. Clin Podiatr Med Surg 2004;21(1):1–15.

[13] Roukis TS, Landsman AS. Salvage of the first ray in a diabetic patient with osteomyelitis. J Am Podiatr Med Assoc 2004;94(5):492–8.

ELSEVIER
SAUNDERS

Clin Podiatr Med Surg
25 (2008) 763–766

CLINICS IN
PODIATRIC
MEDICINE AND
SURGERY

Index

Note: Page numbers of article titles are in **boldface** type.

Moving?

Make sure your subscription moves with you!

To notify us of your new address, find your **Clinics Account Number** (located on your mailing label above your name), and contact customer service at:

E-mail: elspcs@elsevier.com

800-654-2452 (subscribers in the U.S. & Canada)
1-407-563-6020 (subscribers outside of the U.S. & Canada)

Fax number: 407-363-9661

Elsevier Periodicals Customer Service
6277 Sea Harbor Drive
Orlando, FL 32887-4800

*To ensure uninterrupted delivery of your subscription, please notify us at least 4 weeks in advance of move.

United States Postal Service

Statement of Ownership, Management, and Circulation
(All Periodicals Publications Except Requestor Publications)

1. Publication Title
Clinics in Podiatric Medicine & Surgery

2. Publication Number
0 0 0 _ 7 7 0 7

3. Filing Date
9/15/08

4. Issue Frequency
Jan, Apr, Jul, Oct

5. Number of Issues Published Annually
4

6. Annual Subscription Price
$208.00

7. Complete Mailing Address of Known Office of Publication *(Not printer) (Street, city, county, state, and ZIP+4)*

Elsevier Inc.
360 Park Avenue South
New York, NY 10010-1710

Contact Person
Stephen Bushing

Telephone *(Include area code)*
215-239-3688

8. Complete Mailing Address of Headquarters or General Business Office of Publisher *(Not printer)*

Elsevier Inc., 360 Park Avenue South, New York, NY 10010-1710

9. Full Names and Complete Mailing Addresses of Publisher, Editor, and Managing Editor *(Do not leave blank)*

Publisher *(Name and complete mailing address)*

John Schrefer , Elsevier, Inc., 1600 John F. Kennedy Blvd. Suite 1800, Philadelphia, PA 19103-2899

Editor *(Name and complete mailing address)*

Patrick Manley, Elsevier, Inc., 1600 John F. Kennedy Blvd. Suite 1800, Philadelphia, PA 19103-2899

Managing Editor *(Name and complete mailing address)*

Catherine Bewick, Elsevier, Inc., 1600 John F. Kennedy Blvd. Suite 1800, Philadelphia, PA 19103-2899

10. Owner *(Do not leave blank. If the publication is owned by a corporation, give the name and address of the corporation immediately followed by the names and addresses of all stockholders owning or holding 1 percent or more of the total amount of stock. If not owned by a corporation, give the names and addresses of the individual owners. If owned by a partnership or other unincorporated firm, give its name and address as well as those of each individual owner. If the publication is published by a nonprofit organization, give its name and address.)*

Full Name	Complete Mailing Address
Wholly owned subsidiary of	4520 East-West Highway
Reed/Elsevier, US holdings	Bethesda, MD 20814

11. Known Bondholders, Mortgagees, and Other Security Holders Owning or Holding 1 Percent or More of Total Amount of Bonds, Mortgages, or Other Securities. If none, check box. ☐ None

Full Name	Complete Mailing Address
N/A	

12. Tax Status *(For completion by nonprofit organizations authorized to mail at nonprofit rates) (Check one)*
The purpose, function, and nonprofit status of this organization and the exempt status for federal income tax purposes:
☐ Has Not Changed During Preceding 12 Months
☐ Has Changed During Preceding 12 Months *(Publisher must submit explanation of change with this statement)*

PS Form 3526, September 2006 (Page 1 of 3 (Instructions Page 3)) PSN 7530-01-000-9931 PRIVACY NOTICE: See our Privacy policy in www.usps.com

---

13. Publication Title
Clinics in Podiatric Medicine & Surgery

14. Issue Date for Circulation Data Below
July 2008

15. Extent and Nature of Circulation			**Average No. Copies Each Issue During Preceding 12 Months**	**No. Copies of Single Issue Published Nearest to Filing Date**
a. Total Number of Copies *(Net press run)*			1625	1600
b. Paid Circulation (By Mail and Outside the Mail)	(1)	Mailed Outside-County Paid Subscriptions Stated on PS Form 3541. *(Include paid distribution above nominal rate, advertiser's proof copies, and exchange copies)*	954	908
	(2)	Mailed In-County Paid Subscriptions Stated on PS Form 3541 *(Include paid distribution above nominal rate, advertiser's proof copies, and exchange copies)*		
	(3)	Paid Distribution Outside the Mails Including Sales Through Dealers and Carriers, Street Vendors, Counter Sales, and Other Paid Distribution Outside USPS®	64	55
	(4)	Paid Distribution by Other Classes Mailed Through the USPS (e.g. First-Class Mail®)		
c. Total Paid Distribution *(Sum of 15b (1), (2), (3), and (4))*		►	1018	963
d. Free or Nominal Rate Distribution (By Mail and Outside the Mail)	(1)	Free or Nominal Rate Outside-County Copies Included on PS Form 3541	77	119
	(2)	Free or Nominal Rate In-County Copies Included on PS Form 3541		
	(3)	Free or Nominal Rate Copies Mailed at Other Classes Mailed Through the USPS (e.g. First-Class Mail)		
	(4)	Free or Nominal Rate Distribution Outside the Mail (Carriers or other means)		
e. Total Free or Nominal Rate Distribution *(Sum of 15d (1), (2), (3) and (4))*		►	77	119
f. Total Distribution *(Sum of 15c and 15e)*		►	1095	1082
g. Copies not Distributed *(See instructions to publishers #4 (page #3))*		►	530	518
h. Total *(Sum of 15f and g)*		►	1625	1600
i. Percent Paid *(15c divided by 15f times 100)*		►	92.97%	89.00%

16. Publication of Statement of Ownership
☐ If the publication is a general publication, publication of this statement is required. Will be printed in the **October 2008** issue of this publication.   ☐ Publication not required

17. Signature and Title of Editor, Publisher, Business Manager, or Owner

[signature]

Rancor — Executive Director of Subscription Services   September 15, 2008

I certify that all information furnished on this form is true and complete. I understand that anyone who furnishes false or misleading information on this form or who omits material or information requested on the form may be subject to criminal sanctions (including fines and imprisonment) and/or civil sanctions (including civil penalties).

PS Form 3526, September 2006 (Page 2 of 3)

Printed and bound by CPI Group (UK) Ltd, Croydon, CR0 4YY

08/06/2025

01896870-0005